The How of Ow

Everyday Self-Care and the Art of Pain Relief

by Wanda Jean Swenson, PT

Phoenix Century Press
P.O. Box 1792
Sausalito, CA 94966

www.phoenixcenturypress.com

Neither the author nor the publisher is engaged in rendering professional advice or services to the individual reader. The ideas, procedures, and suggestions contained in this book are not intended as a substitute for consulting with your physician. All matters regarding your health require medical supervision. Neither the author nor the publisher shall be liable for any loss or damage allegedly arising from any information or suggestion in this book.

The How of Ow

Everyday Self-Care
and the Art of Pain Relief

by Wanda Jean Swenson, PT

ISBN-13: 978-0-9600691-0-1
www.thehowofow.com

Interior design and illustrations by Gary Newman
Cover design by Wanda Swenson and Gary Newman

Printed in the United States of America

In Memory of

Keiko Fukuda

"Be strong, be gentle, be beautiful."

9th dan Kodokan
10th dan USA Judo/US Judo Federation

1913-2013

TABLE OF CONTENTS

PART FOUR

Introduction

L earning from experience is something we all can do. As a physical therapist, perhaps I've taken this to an extreme. Once I took an inventory of all my injuries and realized I'd had some degree of strain, pain, or traumatic injury to every joint in my body! I'm not recommending this particularly for every budding physical therapist, but I must say, it's worked for me.

Over 30 years working as a physical therapist, I saw many people with injuries similar to my own. I'd see them weeks, and sometimes months or years, after they'd occurred. By that time, simple strains and pains had often become more complicated pain conditions. I began to think "Wouldn't it be great to have a book that describes how a physical therapist approaches her own self-care, and avoid the delay of early treatment?"

However, what really inspired me to sit down and write, was not my timely recovery from so many injuries and strains, but rather my eventual recovery from chronic back pain that didn't improve with my standard PT practices. This is when I stumbled upon the idea, that I later named Postural Isometric Lengthening (PIL), which is a prominent theme, found throughout these pages.

Years ago, I had a very mild strain in my back, which I ignored. We all make mistakes! Then, I proceeded to severely strain the same

This Book Can Help the Reader:

- Learn about the nature of pain and the timeline of healing. Not knowing what to do or how long it will take to recover from injury can lead to strong emotional reactions to pain. Fear, anxiety, and depression add to the sensation of pain. The current opioid epidemic and the use of prescription opioids for orthopedic pain reflect this lack of understanding about the psychology of pain.
- Understand that taking medications or going to health care practitioners (physical therapists, chiropractors, massage therapists, etc.) can't completely fix a problem. We need to take personal responsibility. Self-care and using practical mindfulness is the basis of *The How of Ow*.
- Develop awareness that poor body mechanics makes us weaker and hinders recovery. Using good body mechanics with everyday activities makes us stronger and more flexible and gives us pain relief.
- Learn how to strengthen and heal deeper muscles that have been weakened by injury. These are the deep muscles of the neck, low back, shoulders, and hips. Using good body mechanics and doing simple postures and isometric exercise during the day uses these muscles and strengthens them.
- Gain awareness that stretching sore muscles without strengthening them is ineffective for pain relief. People often think they just need to "stretch out" something for pain. Over stretching painful areas often increases our sensitivity to pain making our perception of pain worse.
- Understand that the body compensates for limited movement in one area by having more movement in another—explaining how chronic pain conditions "spread" to other parts of the body. Regaining movement of painful joints and flexibility of surrounding muscles relieves stress and strain in other parts of the body.

area working in my yard and shoveling heavy clay. I got myself to the house slowly—the only way I could move—with a spasm in my left lower back. I did all the typical self-care physical therapy I knew to do. I lay down, used ice, took an anti-inflammatory, and did basic lumbar spine range of motion and strengthening exercises. I was extra careful with posture and body mechanics. I managed my pain, but for months I would still get a spasm in my back by the end of the day at work. I would have to stretch or sit down. If I had the time I'd use some heat on it. I continued to do spinal stabilization strengthening exercises using equipment in our clinic (a Pilates reformer) and would take lots of walks. At home I'd have to take more breaks and lie down after working in the garden. I had bodywork done (PT manual therapy, cranio-sacral and massage therapy) with some improvement. But every afternoon the spasm would return.

I decided to get an X-ray to see how bad my back looked. I knew I had degenerative conditions in my spine, but I was shocked to see my X-ray. I have one of the worst looking spines I've ever seen! (A severe degenerative lumbar scoliosis—bad arthritis with a sideways curve.) I began to think that I might just have to lie down every afternoon the way my grandmother (whom I resemble) did to "rest" her back.

After months of this I went on a daylong silent meditation retreat. One hour of sitting meditation alternating with one hour of walking meditation. I knew sitting on the floor would be too hard for me, so I chose a chair. I was fine in the morning, but by afternoon my back started to go into spasm. I opened my eyes and looked at the people sitting on the floor in front of me. More than half of them were wiggling around, stretching overhead, bending forward, and twisting. All the things I usually would do when my back was in spasm just to get some relief.

Then the inspiration hit me. "I'm not going to do that. I'm going to do the exact opposite of that." I sat as tall as I could to lengthen my trunk, tighten my buttocks, and pull my belly in towards my spine (as in the lumbar stabilization strengthening exercise). I further lengthened the back of my neck and pressed my shoulder blades together and down. The final effort was imagining a steel door pushing against me and I was meeting its pressure. In this extreme isometric posture, doing slow diaphragmatic breathing, I had no back pain. I held this pose for a minute or longer and then relaxed. The pain came back, but not as bad as before. I kept doing this posture and then relaxing, managing the pain quite well.

The next day I got through the afternoon pain free, and the spasm never returned! Since then, when I occasionally have some back pain—or any spinal pain—I immediately do this posture (PIL) in standing, sitting, or while walking and get relief.

I later found out that I hadn't discovered anything new. In fact, this posture is several thousand years old and very similar to Banda yoga, a form of yoga that emphasizes an "internal locking", or isometric strengthening, with spinal lengthening.

In this book you'll read about personal and and clinical experiences that demonstrate the effectiveness of self-care principles. Illustrations with clear instruction explain simple ways to immediately strengthen and lengthen the spine during daily activities (PIL, Postural Isometric Lengthening) for the early onset of any spinal (neck, mid back, or low back) strain and for strains to areas with muscular connection to the spine (TMJ, shoulders, hips). It describes ways to prevent common strains, as well as how to regain strength and return to normal mobility through the use of good body mechanics. Sidebars give additional information about muscles, joints, and their surrounding soft tissues, as well as other associated topics.

Techniques for returning to normal balance and walking after painful conditions or prolonged bed rest are given. Also provided are head-to-toe methods for recovering from nerve pain as well as specific joint and muscle injuries.

There's a lot of information here. The best way to get the most out of it is to read through it initially, and then re-read one part at a time.

Continue to refer to it until the concepts become second nature and use it as a reference book when any problems arise.

Ideally, these tools are used consistently during work or play, while sitting or driving, in bed before sleep, and after waking. You will learn how to reduce the risk of developing—or begin to recover from—chronic pain conditions.

The How of Ow shows you that everyday self-care reduces stress and can become a relaxing and rejuvenating part of daily life. The "art" of pain relief is the practice of creatively applying these skills from moment to moment.

PART ONE

Chapter 1

Now This Won't Hurt a Bit
Misconceptions About Pain

A man in his early forties winced as he stood up awkwardly from the chair in the waiting room, and began to walk slowly towards me, bent forward. In my treatment room he told me that he woke up with low back pain a few months before and really didn't know what had caused it. His doctor had started giving him pain medications, which had helped at first, but as time went on he wasn't getting the same relief as he had initially. Now his pain was even worse than it had been. He couldn't take any more time off work so he wanted the doctor to increase his pain medication or give him something stronger. The doctor told him that he had to try physical therapy first before he would increase his meds. He said to me "I don't really need to be here, but I have to so I can get my pain meds increased."

We all experience pain from time to time. Some of us experience pain, to varying degrees, everyday. There are times we know what caused our pain, and there are other times we can't make sense of it. Most of us wish that feeling good could last forever and that pain would go away immediately.

Unfortunately, pain doesn't work that way. Even if we know exactly what we did that caused our pain and how to recover from it, we still experience pain. It goes away as the injury heals, or the arthritic flare up calms down. If we don't know why arthritic pain has flared up and how to recover from it, or what to do to recover from any injury—whether we know what caused it or not—we can often experience pain for longer periods of time. This is known as chronic pain.

Most people associate pain with injury and assume with chronic pain—pain lasting anywhere from over two weeks to 2-3 months or longer, well beyond the timeline of healing for the severity of the injury—that they are still injured somehow. Minor and moderately painful conditions—from arthritis, muscle strains, or joint sprains—can cause us to think something needs to be protected, like a more severe traumatic injury or flare up. Or we might think we need to power through pain, leaving us feeling even worse. Better yet, we just hope that we'll wake up one morning and the pain will be gone.

Timeline of Healing

- Minor painful conditions* heal and become progressively less sensitive in 1-3 days.
- Moderate painful conditions heal and become progressively less sensitive in 7-14 days.
- Severe painful conditions can heal, or may need surgical intervention and become progressively less sensitive in 2-3 months or up to six months to a year or longer. Some severe conditions can leave us with chronic pain, but our quality of life is improved with less focus on the pain. Pain reduction — less severe pain or intermittent pain—should be experienced when good self-care is used.

---

* Painful conditions include injury and acute inflammation of muscle strains, joint sprains, spinal discs and nerve pain as well as flare-ups of chronic conditions like arthritis, degenerative disc disease, and spinal stenosis.

In recent years it's common to have pain medications prescribed if we go to a doctor for painful orthopedic conditions. Often this is what patients want—"Doctor, give me something for my pain!"—which in part has led us into the current opioid epidemic. My colleagues and I became aware of the dangerous practice of over-prescribing opiates (Codeine, Fentanyl, Hydrocodone, Oxycodone) for orthopedic pains in the early 2000's, as we saw Methadone listed in our patient's medications, being used to get them off prescribed opiates.

We've mistakenly been given the impression that we shouldn't ever have to feel pain, but we haven't been educated about what pain is or how it works. We're just told that the pills will help.

But do they help? Well, they can be great for acute pain. We're often given anti-inflammatory medications and muscle relaxants along with analgesic (pain) medication for recovery from acute painful conditions or surgery. Pain medications act on the brain to reduce our perception of pain, dulling the sensation.* They can help us to sleep more comfortably and move more easily while we're healing. That's great for a while, but if we haven't been progressively getting more active using good self-care to regain strength and flexibility in this early stage, the pain is there again when we stop taking the pills. The healed injury or arthritic joints that haven't been moved or strengthened leave us with joint stiffness, muscle spasm, and weakness, and medications can't help with that. "Hi!" the pain will yell. "I'm back! Did you miss me?"

Then we go back to the doctor and say, "Hey, these drugs aren't working anymore. I need something stronger!" In recent years, it hasn't been uncommon for a doctor to increase dosages or the strength of medications for longer periods of time.

What are the risks and effects of long-term opioid use? They include poor sleep (often a contributing factor to chronic pain), poor mood, fatigue, constipation, slowed cognition as well as worsening pain—the very thing we thought we were treating! And this can go on until we develop drug tolerance (the drug loses effectiveness), dependence, or worse—an

---

* Volkow N, McLellan AT, *Opioid abuse in chronic pain – misconceptions and mitigation strategies.* New England Journal of Medicine 2016; 3-14: 1253-1263.

How Use of Opiates Has Changed

Long before I was even thinking of becoming a PT, I had a back strain so severe that I went to an emergency room. That was in the 1970s— a time when we had to beg for pain meds. Admittedly, I did beg for pain meds. I took them for a day or two, went to a chiropractor and got back to work.

But in the 1990's an opioid, Oxycontin, was promoted by the pharmaceutical industry to medical professionals as being non-addictive due to its time-released component. It turned out Oxycontin was addictive, but at that time doctors risked poor performance evaluations from patients and peers if they didn't adequately treat pain.[*] The increase in marketing for these drugs and a general acceptance in society of their use for orthopedic conditions had patients demanding it for neck and back pain.[†]

Instead of getting better during those two weeks while the prescription lasted, people would just take the drugs and not know what to do for their own recovery. They'd run out of pain pills, the pain would still be there, and doctors often continued to prescribe more pain meds.

This trend is beginning to turn around as pharmaceutical companies and their distributors are being sued and the national spotlight is on the opioid epidemic.[‡§] Drug overdoses on prescription medication have increased with an associated five-fold increase in prescription overdose deaths from 1999 to 2017.[¶] And there is the alarmingly frequent shift from prescription opioids to heroin, since it often is cheaper and more available.[**]

---

[*]   Mandell BF. *The fifth vital sign: A complex story of politics and patient care.* Cleveland Clinic Journal of Medicine. 2016 June; 83(6):400-401.

[†]   This is not to suggest that opioids shouldn't be prescribed for end of life care or cancer pain, and initially after surgery or acute severe injury. Having pain-relieving medications can be a blessing when used appropriately.

[‡]   Center for Disease Control and Prevention. *CDC guideline for prescribing opioids for chronic pain* – United States, 2016. Morbidity Mortality Weekly Report. 2016;65(1).

[§]   Stempel J; Raymond N. *First Criminal Charges in Opioid Epidemic: Rochester Turned a Blind Eye,* US Says. Reuters, April 23, 2019.

[¶]   Center for Disease Control and Prevention. *2018 Annual Surveillance Report of Drug-Related Risks and Outcomes* – United States. Surveillance Special Report 2.

[**] *Pain Management and the Opioid Epidemic; Balancing Societal and Individual Benefits and Risk of Opioid Use.* National Academies of Science, Engineering and Medicine; Health and Medicine Division. Committee on Pain Management and Regulatory Strategies to Address Prescription Opioid Abuse; Phillips JK, Ford MA, Bonnie RJ editors.

addiction to the drugs. The cycle goes on and on—more pain, more drugs, more pain. It's pretty clear that prolonged use of opiates is bad news.

Cannabis has been promoted as a pain reliever, but since it's illegal federally, standardization and larger research studies have been limited. Cannabis doesn't have the lethal side effects that opioids have, but it can't help with the underlying muscle weakness and joint stiffness, or negative mindset associated with chronic pain.

Then there's that good stiff drink after a long day. We might start needing a drink in the middle of the day, or even in the morning. Although legal, alcohol has lots of side effects on par with the opioids. When alcohol is combined with anti-inflammatory drugs or analgesics, it tends to compound the side effects.*

All in the name of pain relief. But what do we know about pain? We know that pain is a purely subjective experience. Even the most empathetic person can't feel someone else's pain. We can't take out the pain-o-meter and measure how much pain someone is having. We often go

---

* Darnall, Beth, PhD. *Less Pain Fewer Pills: Avoid the Dangers of Prescription Opioids and Gain Control Over Chronic Pain.* Bull Publishing Company, 2014.

Pain Tolerance

A lot of things can affect our sense of pain. As individuals, we all have lower or higher tolerance to pain. When we're in a situation where we need to be taking pain medications, people with low pain tolerance may have a harder time getting off opioid medication. Lower pain tolerance has been associated with early childhood trauma and PTSD.* Endogenous opioids are produced naturally in our body, to suppress the sensation of pain. This is why opiate drugs are effective. Our bodies have receptor sites for an opiate to fit into—like a neuro-chemical lock and key mechanism. When we take opioid medications our body's neuro-chemical production of opioids decreases and we become more sensitive, resulting in a lower tolerance to pain. This is another reason why limiting opiates to short term use is critical.

---

* Darnall, Beth, PhD. *Less Pain Fewer Pills: Avoid the Dangers of Prescription Opioids and Gain Control Over Chronic Pain.* Bull Publishing Company, 2014.

to a doctor because we're having pain. We want to get it diagnosed and treated. Not having a pain-o-meter, doctors depend on recognizing the area of pain—directly at the site of the problem or referred from another area of the body. Then they use diagnostic tools—physical examination, X-ray, MRI, etc.—to make a diagnosis. They also use pain scales (see sidebar). Pain is a clue about where and what a problem is. Pain from a twisted ankle or broken leg makes the search for a diagnosis pretty obvious and we have tools to see if a bone is broken. Or complaints like " It hurts when I do this" can also be a good clue for a doctor's diagnosis or a physical therapist's assessment of a problem.

In that perfect world where pain is brief and feeling good lasts forever, that would be that. We have a problem and we go to someone and they fix our body for us. Or we're given a pill for pain and all is well. No need to know what to do for ourselves or to understand anything about pain.

Unfortunately, this is not how painful conditions or how our minds and bodies work.

Pain Scales

In order to objectify pain, allowing a person to communicate the level of pain they're feeling to someone else—including pain researchers—pain scales have been designed. Basically, this is "On a scale of 0-10 rate your pain, 0 being no pain and 10 being the worst pain imaginable."

Another effective pain scale that focuses more on the mind's attention to pain is the *Pain Catastrophizing Scale*. This asks for a response ranging from "not at all" to "all the time" about worrying, feeling overwhelmed, feeling fearful and helpless about pain. Scoring high on this scale is a good predictor for who will develop chronic pain.*

---

* Severijns, R., et al., *Pain catastrophizing predicts pain intensity, disability, and psychological distress independent of the level of physical impairment.* Clinical Journal of Pain, 2001. 17(2): p. 165-72.

Reminder

Chronic pain is associated with poor self-care in the early stages of recovery.*† Our joints, muscles, and nerves (which give our brains the message of pain) depend on movement for their health. By not moving early in our recovery, everything becomes even more painful when we do try to move. This begins the dangerous cycle of thinking that pain equals injury and that movement must be a bad thing. There is an appropriate time to rest and protect an injury— giving us time to heal. We move slower and take more breaks. We take the time to lie down when we can. This is known as "graded exposure"—gradually developing tolerance to our usual pursuits by starting movement and activity slowly and then building up.

We often take some kind of medications—anti-inflammatory (to reduce pain and swelling) or analgesic drugs (to reduce pain). Initially, we might use ice on a swollen joint and wrap it up to prevent excessive swelling. We can use a cane or a crutch to be able to walk and not put full weight on an injured leg, or wear a sling to support an injured arm. After a car accident, we might feel much better wearing a neck brace or an elastic support for the low back. These are all good initial self-care actions. But when we don't know what to do after this initial acute stage, we often continue this protective phase way too long.

---

* Institute for Brain Potential Seminar: *Psychological Approaches to Managing Pain*. Presented by Darnall B, PhD Clinical Associate Professor in the Department of Anesthesiology, Perioperative, and Pain Medicine at Stanford University.

† Arnold E, LaBarrie J, DaSilva L, Patti M, Goode A, Clewly D. *The impact of timing of physical therapy for acute low back pain on health services utilization: A systematic review*. Archives of Physical Medicine and Rehabilitation; 2019, Jan 23.

Chapter 2

Everything You Ever Wanted to Know About Pain but Were Afraid to Ask

Pain Science

*F*ew people come in to see a doctor or physical therapist wanting to understand the nature of pain. We want it to be like going to a car mechanic. We don't want to know about how the check engine light came on. "Please, just fix the car." But our bodies are different than our cars. We do need to know something about how pain works.

The International Association of the Study of Pain (IASP) gives us the following definition of pain:

Pain is an unpleasant sensory and emotional experience associated with actual or potential tissue damage, or described in terms of such damage.

To begin to change our understanding of pain we need to appreciate two important concepts in this definition:

1. Pain is a sensory experience.
2. Pain is an emotional experience.

Let's first look at the "sensory experience" of pain. This part may not be too surprising, as we all know that we "feel" pain, and physically feeling something is a sensation. But what might not be appreciated is that all body sensations are processed in the brain via the spinal cord. We might think that the pain in a toe after it's been stubbed into a coffee table leg is in the toe, but technically what is felt is in the brain. Sensory nerves from the toe travel up the spinal cord to sensory areas of the brain. We only feel pain once the message has reached the brain.

Yes, the toe may be sprained or scraped, some actual tissue damage may have occurred, but we wouldn't know about it if the brain wasn't giving us the message of pain. Think of having a completely numb foot—like being given a shot of Novocain—and then banging a toe. The toe still gets damaged, but we don't feel the pain if we don't have functioning sensory nerves in the toe getting the message up to the brain.

On the other hand, we don't even have to have a toe to feel pain in it. Phantom pain is a common, but not well understood, condition of people who have had amputations and yet feel considerable pain in the missing limb.

Chronic pain is associated with an injury that has healed. We're still having the sensation of pain in a certain area, but there is no longer any tissue damage.

The next part of this definition to appreciate is that pain is an "emotional experience." As with sensation, emotions and memories

Pain Receptors

Pain receptors from skin, bones, and joints can be closed by use of local anesthetic so we don't feel pain in that area. Think of the use of Novocain when going to the dentist. These receptors are closed and we become numb. Conversely, a bite from a stingray, one of the most painful conditions experienced, keeps these receptors opened. Pain receptors are also more active when we have the flu. That's why we just hurt all over and often any injury we have will feel worse. These receptors are more active when we become "hypersensitive" with chronic pain.

are processed in the brain, in the amygdala and hippocampus. Cussing and yelling after we've banged a toe on that coffee table leg is certainly emotional and many of us can't control that reaction. That's a normal immediate reaction. But what happens long after that initial sensation of acute pain has subsided and we're still having an emotional reaction to lingering pain?

Research into the psychology of pain suggests that everything that affects our nervous system—the brain—affects the perception of pain. This includes emotions, thoughts, beliefs, expectations, and stress. The more the mind focuses on pain in negative ways—thoughts of fear, anxiety, and depression—our pain becomes worse. We might begin to focus on it and catastrophize about it (see Pain Scales, p. 14). We find ourselves wondering "What's wrong with me?" "Will I be able to go back to work?" "Why can't my doctor tell me what's going on?" Our thoughts might frequently be about how bad the pain is, how it might not get better, how it's really messing up our lives and there seems to be nothing we can do about it. We stop doing the things that give us pleasure and just focus on what we can't do because we have pain.

Having unexplained pain increases stress. Stress is associated with our "fight or flight" response via the sympathetic nervous system. We have a protective, hard-wired autonomic pain response to actual or potential tissue damage.

The autonomic nervous system is an involuntarily system that operates without our conscious control. We often aren't even aware of our autonomic response to pain/injury or the threat of pain/injury. The combination of reactions is known as the stress response— or the fight-or-flight response, because it evolved as a survival mechanism, enabling people and other creatures to react quickly to life-threatening situations. This is the action of our sympathetic nervous system. Unconsciously we immediately respond to a threatening situation. It's activated as we're running away from a predator or slamming on the brakes to avoid a car accident.

Unfortunately, the body can also react in the same way to stressors that are not life-threatening, such as traffic jams, work pressure, family difficulties, as well as the pain of banging a toe into that coffee table leg. Physiologically we react the same way to these non-life-threatening events: Heart rate and blood pressure increases, breathing rate increases and becomes more shallow, digestive function decreases, and muscle tension increases.

Stress hormones (cortisol, adrenaline, and others) are released into the blood stream when the sympathetic nervous system is dominant, activating an inflammatory response. This in turn further sensitizes the nervous system and lowers the immune system responses, making it

Placebo and Nocebo Responses

We also have placebo—pain relieving—responses. This is when we've been reassured by a professional, or have a strong belief that something offered to us will reduce or alleviate our pain. It's not that the sensation of pain wasn't real, just that the treatment wasn't what we thought it was. More important is to appreciate how the mind has the ability to override pain. Interestingly, we can also have a nocebo—pain inducing—response if we are given negative expectations. The same substance can be given to test subjects with the only difference being what they are told when it's administered. "This will make your pain worse" or "This will make your pain better." Many subjects will perceive pain according to the suggestion.*

Sometimes we can ignore pain if our life or that of a loved one is threatened. We can perform superhuman feats in the right circumstance. But there are times when the brain is telling us "pain" when there is no danger of further injury to the body—and we focus on it. Chronic pain is no longer telling us about damage. Thoughts and judgments about pain fool us into thinking that there is damage where there isn't any. The pain response has become hypersensitive— giving us too much information when it's not warranted. Focusing on it, being worried about it, changing our lives around it, drawing attention to it, only makes it worse.

---

* Scott, DJ, BS, Stohler, CS, DDS, PhD, Egnatuk, CM, BS, Wang, H, PhD, Koeppe, RA, PhD, Zubieta, JK, MD, PhD. *Placebo and nocebo effects are defined by opposite opioid and dopaminergic responses*, Archive of General Psychiatry/Vol 65 (No. 2), Feb 2008.

easier to succumb to colds or the flu. A hypersensitive nervous system increases our sensation of pain. In severe cases, we can develop allodynia—when even a light touch can feel painful.

It's easy to see that pain is a complicated sensory-emotional experience involving many areas of the brain.

But pain itself, as unpleasant and emotionally charged as it can be, is not life threatening. With painful conditions, the fight or flight response doesn't help at all. Even worse is when we're being less active and more sedentary—in our avoidance of pain—as our muscle tension,

Mindfulness Based Stress Reduction

Since the 1970's mindfulness has been used as a stress reduction technique where western medicine has failed. It draws on meditation techniques and eastern philosophies that observe the nature of the mind and thoughts. It's most useful for stress when applied to everyday life and used briefly throughout the day. MBSR (Mindfulness Based Stress Reduction) is a form of self-help therapy usually taught in groups and commonly used in Pain Clinics.

MBSR has people focus on breathing and observing muscular tension throughout the body. This encourages our parasympathetic nervous system to become dominant, to slow down our breathing and heart rate, lower blood pressure, and relax muscles. Our senses are heightened as we pay attention to sounds and smells or any other sense—taste, vision, touch—that we choose to focus on. We observe thoughts as they come and go.

At least, that's the idea. What usually happens is a thought distracts us. Before we know it, one thought leads to another, and then another. Seconds and minutes pass. We're somewhere else altogether, either lost in the past or the future. We no longer feel the calm of the parasympathetic system. Depending on where our thoughts lead us, our fight or flight system starts to gain the upper hand. We become aware of emotions, the pulse quickens and breathing becomes more shallow. There might be tensing of muscles, clenching of the jaw, pressure in the chest, or increased neck and back pain. When we get lost in thought, we are not aware of the present.

blood pressure, and heart rate increases. Digestive functions may decrease, but we want to eat more. This is right when we need to be getting our strength and flexibility back and returning to our usual activities. Our hyper-arousal stress response is the opposite of what our minds and bodies need to be doing for pain. Reacting negatively and avoiding any movement that might initially cause a slight increase in pain is not what we need to recover from injury or surgery.

Now for some good news! We can easily initiate the opposite autonomic reaction via the parasympathetic nervous system. This is a "relaxation response." Instead of maintaining our fight or flight response, we can take deep breaths, adjust our posture and do movements described in this book as we observe and redirect any negative thoughts we might be having. Yes, we can take yoga or tai chi classes, but we can also do brief, periodic relaxation during our regular daily activities and at night before we go to sleep. We can learn what to do in the present moment for early and immediate self-care for relieving a painful condition.

This is the essence of physical therapy. As physical therapists we reassure our patients that the pain of recovery does not equal injury or harm. Then we redirect the emotional focus away from pain. Awareness of breathing is the first approach to relaxation and awareness of the present moment. Then attention can be directed to habits, how we move, sit, stand, work, and play. We teach the specific movements and strengthening needed to hasten recovery.

Applying mindfulness, or awareness, to our everyday activities allows us to observe our sensations of pain and our emotional thoughts and judgments about pain. We take deep breaths and change our posture and the way we move, encouraging our bodies to heal and relieve pain. This is the essence of *The How Of Ow*.

Reminder

For more complicated and difficult problems concerning stress and related pain conditions—especially if there's a history of PTSD or childhood trauma—a psychotherapist who treats chronic pain can help. Consider this instead of accepting more pain medication from your doctor: Ask for a referral to a psychotherapist. Or pick up a book on the subject—see references (pp. 241-242). It's been suggested that perhaps psychotherapy should be the first strategy, not the last, for chronic pain conditions.

Chapter 3

The Burned Foot Story

Experience Is the Greatest Teacher of All

*E*arly in my practice I worked in the outpatient department of a university hospital. I saw a man who had burned his right lower leg and foot with hot cooking oil, causing a second-degree burn (blistered skin). After six months his skin had healed, but the pain was still unbearable.

I've told this story many times to people experiencing the fear, or negative emotional response, to the unpleasant sensation of pain when first moving after a strain, injury, or surgery. It shows how focusing on recovery—and not on the pain itself—can have dramatic results.

The patient suffered from complex regional pain syndrome, an uncommon type of severe chronic pain affecting the autonomic nervous system. It usually affects an arm or a leg, and develops after an injury has healed with pain out of proportion to the severity of the initial injury.

Trying to avoid additional pain, we think that rest will help and we'll wake up one morning pain free. But it turns out to be the exact opposite. Initially movement does cause more pain. If we avoid movement, decreased blood flow and the loss of strength and flexibility perpetuate the severity of the pain.

The man with the burned foot couldn't tolerate the opiate drugs the doctors had offered him. He was subsequently referred to a neurosurgeon for a neural ablation surgery, which would sever sensory areas of the brain that related to his right foot and lower leg. Needless to say, it was a procedure that offered significant risk and only modest hope for success. He was searching for an alternative. He asked his surgeon if he could see a physical therapist who might be able to help him walk again. He wanted to try being more active in his health care and of course wanted to avoid having the recommended, and terrifying, brain surgery.

He came to the appointment wearing pants with the right leg rolled up, his bare foot pointing downward. He walked by leaning sideways on a crutch under his left arm and hopping forward on his left foot. The skin on his right leg and foot was shiny and hairless, typical of this condition.

It wouldn't seem that he'd caught a break coming to see a PT who had just completed her studies. I did have the training about "desensitizing" a painful extremity by starting slowly with movement and gradually increasing activity (graded exposure) but having had my own second degree burn injury on the bottom of my foot a few years earlier gave me the confidence I needed to work with him.

After hearing his story I said, "A similar thing happened to my foot. It hurt like hell. The pain got better the more I was able to move it and put weight on it. The pain you're having now is not telling you about injury. Your injury, the burn, has healed. You're feeling pain that has nothing to do with injuring yourself more."

He was a little skeptical, but highly motivated, and motivation tops skepticism every time. I coaxed him into putting his leg in a whirlpool of warm water and moving his ankle a little at a time, taking slow, deep breaths. I suggested that he use warm compresses and footbaths at home, gently massaging his foot and leg with a body lotion. He progressed by moving his ankle and knee more, and sitting in a chair with his foot on the floor. Soon he was able to stand with his foot on the floor and to slowly shift weight onto his painful leg. Later on, he was doing heel lifts, partial squats, and balancing on his injured leg.

Of course it was painful, but the pain lessened as he became more active. The biggest change was that he was no longer focused on his pain. He was engaged in the present by doing something about his leg. Now he was focusing on what he was doing and not just the looping pain message that his brain was sending him. He wasn't reacting emotionally, negatively, to the pain.

It was an amazing experience for me as a new therapist to see him come into the office after a couple of weeks of treatment, wearing a shoe on his right foot and walking fairly normally! Not completely better, but getting there.

The beauty of this was that a simple physical self-care treatment, along with his more powerful change of mind, enabled him to overcome the severely debilitating pain he had experienced. He became responsible for his own recovery.

I've used this story as a dramatic example of what happens when we avoid pain and confuse feeling pain with injury. Being immobilized often is needed to allow an injury to heal. A leg is placed in a cast after breaking a bone to allow the bone to mend back together. After surgeries we often need to avoid movement to allow the surgical site to heal. Full movement is often limited after any type of strain to our muscles or sprain to a joint.

Healthy nerves are described as being bloodthirsty (the brain is 2% of the body mass and uses 20% of the oxygen supply) and movement is how they get a good blood supply. They need the oxygen delivered through circulation for their health and normal function. Many of us have experienced a numb arm if we have leaned on it for too long, decreasing circulation to the nerves supplying function to our hand. And what do we do to get it back to normal? We move, by shaking the hand and arm around or making a fist and then stretching it out get blood back into those nerves and tissues.

Chronic lack of blood flow, as in medical conditions like diabetes, causes sensory nerve damage and the associated abnormal sensations of diabetic neuropathy (pins and needles or pain) for many people suffering with this condition. In healthy individuals without chronic problems with circulation, immobilization causes a temporary decrease in circulation to smaller blood vessels, which makes our nerves and tissues—skin, tendons, muscles, joints—less healthy. When we first start moving we feel the unpleasant—or in this case a temporary abnormal—sensation of pain. But this kind of pain does not equal harm.

Reminder

As we move and get our strength back, our nerves become normal again. The pain improves and goes away.

Ironically, what we don't know about pain can hurt us.

SUMMARY OF PART ONE

1. Experiencing pain is a normal part of life. Our emotional reaction and focus on it can make it worse by keeping us from doing what we need to do to recover.

2. Moving slowly and restoring normal movement and strength with effective early self-care will hasten recovery and lessen pain.

3. There are predictable timelines to healing. Pain is tolerated better when we know how long an injury or pain condition will take to recover—1-3 days for a minor condition; 7-14 days for a moderate condition; 2-3 months for a severe condition; up to 6-12 months or longer for a more complicated severe condition.

4. Opiates for pain relief or orthopedic conditions should be used briefly and cautiously, if at all.

PART TWO

Chapter 4

Gravity: Friend or Foe
Introduction to Postural Isometric Lengthening (PIL)

O *ne day my first patient was a fit woman in her early 60s. She'd been to see her doctor for back pain she was still having weeks after she did a marathon gardening workout. Prior to this she'd only had back pain occasionally and never for this long. Now she found walking difficult and sitting uncomfortable. Sleep was fitful and turning in bed gave her sharp pains. Anti-inflammatory medications helped dull the pain temporarily. The doctor sent her to get X-rays of her lumbar spine.*

She spoke haltingly as she revealed what they had found. "I went back to the doctor and she told me that I have"—she paused for dramatic effect—"degenerative disc disease and degenerative joint disease with degenerative lumbar scoliosis! She said I should just get used to having back pain and that there's nothing we can do about it."

I assured her, "Oh yes, there is."

If we're over a certain age and we have X-rays taken of the spine, a "degenerative" condition will usually show up. It's rare to find a person over 40 who doesn't have some degree of joint wear and tear—mild, moderate, or severe—in the neck and low back.

The good news is that spinal pain is sometimes, but often not, related to X-ray or MRI findings. Since the 1960s many research articles show that osteoarthritis (degenerative joint disease) and degenerative disc disease in the spine do not necessarily relate to having pain.[*][†] Many people with excellent looking X-rays have back pain, and many people with bad looking X-rays, showing osteoarthritis and degenerative disc disease, don't have any pain at all.

It has been a fairly standard practice to take an X-ray of anyone with neck and back pain. Sometimes this is done to rule out other possible medical conditions. With an otherwise clean bill of health, the diagnosis

---

*   Witt I , Vertergaard A, Rosenklit A. *A comparative analysis of X-ray findings of the lumbar spine with and without lumbar pain.* Spine Journal, April 1984.

†   Torgerson WR, Dotter WE. *Comparative roentgenographic study of the asymptomatic and symptomatic lumbar spine.* Journal of Bone and Joint Surgery (Am), 1976.

Spinal Degeneration

Degenerative conditions of the spine as we age are normal. Degenerative disc disease is the normal wear and tear and compression of the discs— fibrous cartilage and ligamentous tissue firmly attached between the vertebrae. Intervertebral disc compression helps explain why a lot of us lose height as we age. Degenerative joint disease is the same as osteoarthritis. It's the normal wear and tear of joint surfaces. Spinal stenosis is the narrowing of the spaces between the vertebrae where nerve roots exit.

Degenerative lumbar scoliosis is a diagnosis that we'll probably be hearing more of as the baby boomer population ages. It's not an uncommon condition but has only been given as a diagnosis in recent years.

Degenerative scoliosis is a sideways curve of the lumbar spine seen in people usually older than 40-50. It has the associated osteoarthritis and degenerative disc conditions typical of the aging spine. Postural changes are often seen in standing and walking—bent forward and tilted to the side.

of pain due to degenerative disc disease or osteoarthritis is still often given.

These degenerative conditions do not occur over night. If we didn't have pain a week ago and the back started hurting after getting home from a trip back east or after working too much in the garden, arthritis is not what caused the pain. It's muscle strain or spasm with an underlying degenerative condition of the spine. As research has shown repeatedly, these conditions in themselves do not cause the initial pain. They may cause morning stiffness and less movement in the spine, but acute pain is related more often to muscle strain, spasm, and weakness. Chronic pain can develop due to becoming less active and getting weaker.

One thing's for sure. As we age, more than ever, the body needs to move. We lose water content in soft tissues—muscles, tendons, and ligaments— and in the cartilage of joints. Movement gets the blood flowing, providing oxygen and nutrients to muscles and pushes fluids through the tissues of joints that don't have direct blood supplies. That's why we feel stiff first thing in the morning or after we've just been sitting and haven't

Muscle Spasm

A muscle spasm is a natural protective response of sudden muscle shortening or contraction. Many of us have experienced a "charley horse" in the back of the calves or thighs. These are muscle fibers in spasm. The sudden pain and stiffness really gets our attention and signals that something's wrong. Especially when a spasm occurs in the muscles of the neck or back. It's hard to move at all! Movement becomes limited to initially protect muscles, joints, or nerves. Knowing what to do for a muscle spasm is often key to preventing much worse trouble down the line. Fear of moving in a way that will trigger a muscle spasm causes us to move in awkward ways, which in turn, gives us more problems.

Muscles will also go into spasm when a bone has been broken or a joint badly injured. If we've experienced a traumatic, high speed, high impact injury with the possibility of broken bones or severe joint injury, we should seek medical attention.

Note: A lesser degree of muscle spasm also occurs in milder joint injuries and muscle strains.

moved for a while. It's why everything can feel better after we get up and walk around. Sensory nerves heading up to the brain need blood flow, and oxygen in particular, and we get blood flowing more as we move.

What happens that makes movements and postures change so much? Do we just wake up one morning old and decrepit? Some mornings it does feel that way. Or does it happen when we have horrible back pain getting out of that comfy chair we've sat in so many times, and can't straighten up as we stand?

The key difference between people with back pain and those who didn't have pain with degenerative conditions of the spine has been found to be the position of the pelvis.* When the pelvis and sacrum (the lowest part of the spine that sits between the pelvic bones) are tilted forward most people have minimal complaints of pain. If the pelvis is rounded backward—like sitting slumped with the back rounded out—there are more complaints of pain. Trying to walk around with the pelvis rounded backward makes us walk bent forward. It's the caricature of an older posture—a posture that's bent forward and often tilted to the side. Usually there's a need to walk with a cane and eventually a walker as the postural changes progress.

In my early days as a PT, we were trained to instruct people to walk with the pelvis tucked under—flattening the back—for low back pain associated with arthritis and stenosis. Most likely, many of you reading this who have been diagnosed with a degenerative condition of the low back, have been told at some point that this position of a "flat back" is exactly what you need to do. (The thinking was that pain was coming from the compressed joints of the spine and a tucked pelvic position would cause less compression of the joint surfaces and make more space for the nerve roots exiting between vertebrae.) But walking with the pelvis tucked and the low back rounded is not only incredibly awkward and unnatural but further strains the muscles of the low back. Overall, it just doesn't work. But people walk like this because the initial movement of rocking the pelvis forward is painful due to muscle strain and sensitivity of strained

---

*   Han F, Weishi Li, Zhuoran S, Qingwei M, Zhongqiang C. *Sagittal plane analysis of the spine and pelvis in degenerative lumbar scoliosis.* Journal of Orthopedic Surgery, 2017; Vol:25(1)1-6.

tissues—including tendons and ligaments. Not to mention that people don't realize how important regaining this pelvic movement is!

It's no wonder that research looking at pelvic position and degenerative lumbar scoliosis, associated a tucked position of the pelvis with having worse low back pain. The truth of the matter is that with significant degenerative conditions of the low back or after spinal fusion surgery, the lumbar spine is flattened and has lost its lordosis or inward curve. That's not going to change. What can change is the movement and position of the pelvis relative to the spine by encouraging the coordination, movement and flexibility of the muscles surrounding the pelvis.

As always, the first thing that has to change is our attention to, awareness of, and knowledge about strengthening and lengthening the spine. We can choose to not let an emotional reaction to the unpleasant sensation of pain keep us from moving. We can be aware and observe our reaction to pain knowing that any discomfort with slow movement does not equal harm. Take a deep breath—inhale and exhale—and then move.

The goal of any spinal exercise or treatment is to be able to assume a straight lengthened posture, and to be able to arch backwards slightly in standing or in sitting. Many people think they just need to stretch forward more when their neck or back hurts. What works much better initially for any spinal pain, and can be done anywhere, anytime, around anyone, is Postural Isometric Lengthening (PIL).

Isometric Muscle Contraction and Tractioning

Tightening muscles while we're not moving is an isometric contraction. Tractioning is a lengthening of joints, and a common treatment for spinal pain and degenerative conditions. Tractioning is also a common request of folks when they come in to see a PT: "Could you just pull my head off?" And it's what we crave when we need to lie down or flop into that comfy chair. When the force of gravity is more than we can manage, we want to lie down to relieve the pressure.

Postural Isometric Lengthening (PIL) is "active" tractioning—using muscles—to lengthen and strengthen the spine against gravity.

POSTURAL ISOMETRIC LENGTHENING (PIL)

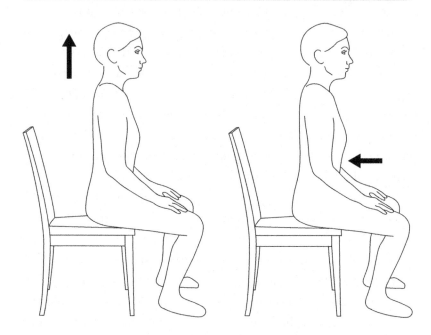

It's best to explain the basic principles of PIL from a sitting position. First, scoot forward to the edge of a seat or move to a higher one. Take a few deep breaths. Slowly, sit as tall as possible. This lengthens the spine (tractioning the spine) and gets the pelvis in a forward position. If this is painful, just relax, slumping slightly, and do it again. Slumping stretches the strained muscles that are in spasm. Take the time to fully lengthen the trunk, sitting tall. Do this a few times if needed. As strained back muscles contract they may initially be painful, but after a few repetitions more blood flows into the muscle and it becomes more comfortable.

Next, hold the lengthened position of the spine and pull the belly in towards the spine as if trying to zip up a pair of pants that are too tight. Hold this position for 5 seconds and continue to breathe naturally, keeping shoulders down. Then relax. The next two chapters give more detailed descriptions of doing PIL in standing and while walking, and "Slump"/ PIL in sitting and in bed.

All the exercises in this book can be done during daily activities, not necessarily at a special exercise time. The art of pain relief becomes the yoga of life. Yoga doesn't have a single definition. Yoga can be described as a conscious connection that allows us to feel and experience a moment more fully, even if that moment is a painful one.

Of course, yoga can be what we do when we go to a yoga class. For many people doing yoga or tai chi, or any mindful exercise is great, but they might not know the advantages of applying those exercises to everyday life. Others would rather just take a walk, dance, play sports, or work in the garden.

Anything can be done mindfully. The body needs attention as we have aches and pains during the day and PIL can be done briefly with any activity. Responding in the moment to muscle strain or joint pain greatly reduces the time it takes to recover.

Reminder

As we age, degenerative conditions of the spine are normal. Chronic pain doesn't have to be. PIL is a simple way to strengthen and lengthen the spine with our everyday activities. These are exercises we always have time for, because whatever we do—there we are. We don't need to make a date to get together with ourselves. We only need awareness of the present and the knowledge about what to do in the moment when we experience pains and strains.

Chapter 5

A PIL that Does Make You Taller
The Yoga of Life

Some people dread going to see a physical therapist for fear they will be judged. So they come in, sit down, and declare, "I have terrible posture!" More often than not, after saying that, they'd sit up straight and tall without any goading from me.

"No," I'd say. "You have beautiful posture. What are you talking about?"

Then they'd admit, "I just straightened up because you were looking at me."

I'd reply, "Well, you still have good posture. Maybe you don't use it much, but your posture's fine."

Whenever we can't tolerate standing, walking, or even sitting—because of back or neck pain (or associated arm and leg pain)—the physical problem is about instability and weakness in the spine.

Think of the spine. It's 24 bones (the vertebrae), plus the fused bones of the sacrum and coccyx (tailbone), stacked on top of each other. It's really easy for these to get knocked down, right? Ligaments (fibrous

soft tissue connecting bones to bones around joints) and the discs (fibrous cartilage and ligaments between the vertebrae) give a degree of
support to the spine. But what really supports the spine—what gives it
stability as we move—are deep abdominal (stomach) muscles working
with the deep muscles in the back of the spine, and deep muscles in
the front of the neck.

Deep muscles are muscles closer to bone. Superficial muscles are the
ones closer to the skin. We can see the superficial muscles on some of us
better than others, depending on how much fat we have under our skin
or how thin our muscles might be. Think of a body builder or pro-wres-
tler types, with the famous "six-pack" of abdominal muscles. Those are
superficial or surface muscles, not the ones that support the spine. When
a body builder or a lean sprinter has a back strain, we can still see those
well-defined muscles. But their deeper muscles are on the blink.

The deep abdominal muscles and deep back muscles are the unsung
heroes, the hidden workers behind the scene. When we've injured the
back—in car accidents, from lifting badly, by getting out of a car awkwardly, by slipping and falling, or slipping and not falling—the strained
deep muscles are not working well together. This is why it's so hard to do
anything when the back has been tweaked badly. Reaching away from
the body or bending forward becomes almost impossible. The superficial
muscles don't hold the spine together like the deep ones do. The superficial
muscles move the spine, but they don't stabilize the individual vertebrae.

Now, I'm not suggesting that we walk through life doing PIL constantly. In fact, not at all! Many people are turned off by a physical
therapist that gives them the impossible task of maintaining some kind
of "perfect" posture all the time. They leave their appointment feeling
defeated by a seemingly unattainable heroic task of constantly having
perfect posture. That's not only impossible, it's not even a good idea!
Bodies like movement—not being stuck in a rigid immobilized position. When the deep muscles are in good shape, we have the ability to
move easily without effort.

The idea is simply to use PIL occasionally during the day and more often if we're having pain. Hold the position for a few seconds and then relax. By rocking the pelvis forward and doing PIL, we're strengthening muscles that have been strained, and lengthening the spine to remove stress on joints. It's even good to slump or bend forward briefly, before or after doing PIL in sitting. This is the essence of good early self-care for the spine.

If we have chronic pain, doing PIL when pain increases turns the focus away from pain. It improves strength and muscle coordination, and begins to relieve symptoms.

If we're not having any spinal pain, doing PIL occasionally while sitting and before standing up is a good way to check that everything's OK with the spine. If we can do Slump/PIL with ease, just carry on with what you're doing!

Deep Stabilizing Abdominal Muscles

There are four layers of abdominal muscles with muscle fibers aligned in different directions. The rectus abdominis muscle is the most superficial, and runs lengthwise to the spine. The internal and external oblique muscles run diagonally in opposite directions. The deepest muscle is the transverse abdominis. Its fibers run horizontally, like a wide internal belt. It attaches to the thoracolumbar fascia, connecting it to the deep back muscles. The deep abdominals and the deep back muscles work together as they support and stabilize the low back, much like wearing a corset or a big wide belt that weight lifters or construction workers use. Pulling the belly in towards the spine contracts the transverse abdominis. Reaching away from the body automatically engages this muscle.

PIL IN SITTING 1

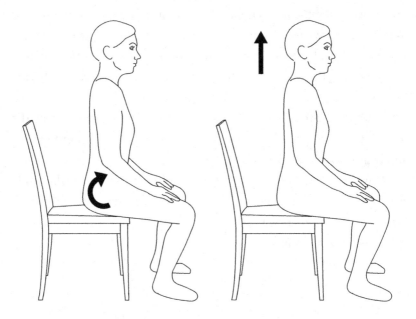

- Sit at the edge of a seat.
- Rock the pelvis forward and lengthen the trunk. Sit as tall as possible, pushing up against gravity.
- Tighten the buttocks.

Note: If there's an excessive arch in the low back (sway back), sitting tall will make the low back arch less.

PIL IN SITTING 2

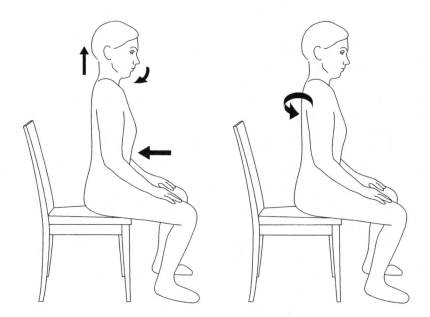

- Tuck in the chin.
- Lengthen the back of the neck.
- Again, sit as tall as possible.
- Pull the belly in towards the spine—just like trying to zip up a pair of pants that are too tight.
- Pull the shoulder blades together and slightly downward. Again, lengthen the back of the neck.
- Check that teeth are apart and the tip of the tongue is on the roof of the mouth—where it rests after saying the word "mine."
- Hold this position and breath slowly and deeply (two second count inhale/three second count exhale) 3-5 times, keeping the belly pulled in towards the spine. Feel the breath expand the lower ribs.

Note: To increase the effect of the isometric strengthening, imagine something pushing the body forward and "push" back into it.

SLUMP/PIL

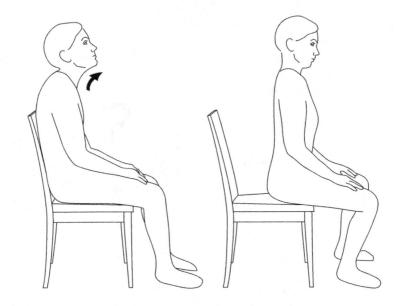

- Relax, letting the back round out and the chin jut forward (an exaggerated slump position). Hold briefly.

Note: If having arm or leg symptoms coming from the spine (p.52), just do PIL and don't do slumped sitting until these symptoms resolve.

- Do slump. Then move slowly into PIL.
- Do this 3-5 times back and forth, moving from an exaggerated slump position into the PIL position (Postural Isometric Lengthening).

UNSUPPORTED PIL SITTING IN CAR SEAT

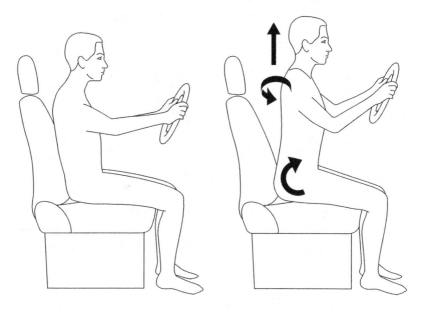

- Scoot the hips back deep into seat.
- Do PIL with the upper back away from the back support of the seat.
- Take a few deep breaths keeping the shoulders down.
- Tuck in the chin and lengthen the back of the neck.
- Repeat 3-5 times until movement is easy and comfortable.
- Relax.

Note: We might feel stiffness in the spine with the first attempt. Continue to do PIL, holding for a few seconds, and then relax until it feels comfortable. For long car or plane rides, holding PIL for up to a minute can be beneficial.

SUPPORTED PIL SITTING IN RECLINED CHAIR

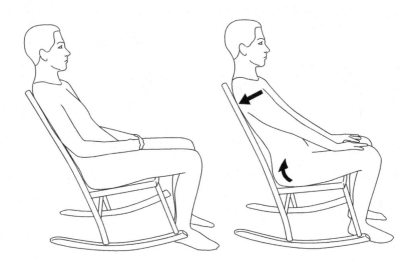

- Scoot the hips back deep in the seat.
- Push the upper back into the backrest and rock the pelvis forward.
- Pinch the shoulder blades together slightly, pull the belly in towards the spine.
- Tuck in the chin and lengthen the back of the neck.
- Hold for a few seconds. Relax.
- Repeat 3-5 times until movement is easy and comfortable.

PIL IN STANDING

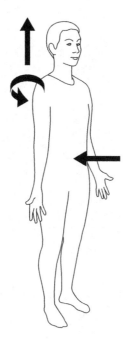

- With feet shoulder width apart, stand as tall as possible.
- Keep the knees slightly relaxed—not locked straight.
- Tuck in the chin and lengthen the back of the neck.
- Pull the belly in towards the spine.
- Tighten the buttocks.
- Have arms at side, palms facing forward. Pinch the shoulder blades slightly together and downward.
- Breathe slowly and deeply, keeping the shoulders down and the belly pulled in towards the spine.
- Again, check to lengthen the back of the neck and stand tall. Check that the teeth are apart and the tongue is resting on the roof of the mouth.
- Hold for 3-5 slow breaths.
- Relax.

BACK EXTENSION IN STANDING

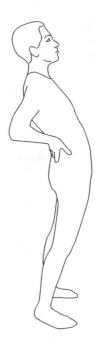

- Stand with the hands supporting the back and slowly arch backwards as far as comfortable.
- Hold 1-3 seconds.
- Repeat 3-5 times.

Note: Good to do PIL with slow walking while taking short steps for back or neck pain, or any leg and arm symptoms coming from the spine.

If having neck pain, maintain the PIL position and try slowly tilting the head side to side (leaning ear towards the shoulder) as far as comfortable. Then try slowly turning the head (looking over the shoulder) as far as comfortable 2-3 times. Stop and move slowly into the other direction if pain increases.

We might find that we're holding the breath as we do PIL. Nothing is going to help us if we're passing out, even with the best intentions of strengthening the spine. The real skill is to learn how to pull in the belly and breathe, at the same time, with ease. Keep practicing!

Get familiar with PIL so it's easy to do whether sitting, driving, or lying down. Then doing it becomes second nature to alleviate pain. It's easy to do PIL standing or sitting for a few seconds after mindlessly slouching. And PIL isn't just key to taking care of neck and back pain. Any strained joints that have muscular connections to the spine (shoulders, jaw, hips), or any referred pain from the spine (headache from the neck, arm or leg pain from the neck or low back), need the spine to be in this lengthened position before we can begin to feel better.

PIL Progression

Sometimes standing has become so uncomfortable that it's really difficult to start doing PIL in standing.

So take a seat, preferably on a firm chair, with feet flat on the floor. Slowly try doing PIL. Maybe it's still not comfortable. That's pretty normal. But remember, not moving is much worse in the long run. So stop when any pain increases and then relax and bend forward, doing the slump stretch. Then slowly do PIL again. Keep going back and forth with Slump/PIL until the PIL position becomes easier and pain lessens.

If things are bad enough, you can apply some ice or heat to the back for 10 to 15 minutes and try doing it again. Doing PIL while sitting with heat on the back or neck is OK, too (page 103).

After being in the PIL position while sitting, stand up keeping the back straight, and stand doing PIL. Try slowly arching backward with hands supporting the back. Do PIL again and start walking slowly, keeping a lengthened spine. Maybe it's just a short walk at first. If you can't stand straight, sit down again and do the same routine.

If you can't do PIL comfortably while sitting, lie down and do it lying on the side (p. 57).

Referred Spinal Pain

Nerves from the neck and low back travel through the arms and legs respectively. Pain coming from the spine, but felt in arms and legs, is often not recognized as spinal pain. It's called "referred pain."

Maybe we're sitting or driving and suddenly have a sharp pain or odd tingling in a leg or an arm. Or maybe it's a stabbing, burning pain in the shoulder blade or arm. And we think, "Wow, I must have strained my leg." Or, "What the heck is wrong with my shoulder blade?"

If we're simply sitting—driving in the car, working at a computer—when this kind of pain comes on, odds are really good that the pain is referred from the spine. Nerves crave oxygen and are asking us to move in the only language they know: Pain, tingling, or numbness.

If we're sitting, we need to scoot the hips back deep in the seat. It's probably sitting slumped for too long that's causing the symptoms in the first place. Hold the PIL position, ideally until the pain goes away. Symptoms will go away if they're coming from the spine. We may need to do a few repetitions—moving in and out of the PIL position—or hold PIL for up to a minute to feel better.

Avoid bending and twisting the spine, or doing prolonged stretches when having referred spinal pain. That will only make the pain worse. Deep rubbing on the area won't help, and may make nerves more sensitive.

Reminder

Doing PIL is just using a lengthened posture as a tool for pain relief and strengthening. It's not a matter of "having" good or bad posture. It's about having awareness to lengthen the spine and to use deep muscles, for pain relief and strengthening.

Chapter 6

Rockin' and Rollin'
PIL and Spinal Exercises to Do in Bed

*O*ne of the funniest moments I had as a PT was when I was
working in a clinic that used curtains instead of doors on the
treatment rooms. I overheard a therapist who was obviously trying
to get her patient to do pelvic rocking (forward and backward movement) while he was lying on his back. She was using every trick in
the book to get him to do the movement. "Try flattening your back
into the table.... Try lifting your low back off my hand.... Imagine
you have a tail and you're tucking your tail between your legs. Push
your stomach downward. Push your stomach upward." This went on
for a while. Then I heard her leafing through the pages of her notes.
With an exasperated sigh she said, "You're married, aren't you?"

Sometimes it's embarrassing to be rocking the pelvis around with
someone we've just met. Or with someone we know but who we don't
have a "pelvis rocking" kind of relationship with. I have a friend who
told me that when he went to a physical therapist, he made her leave
the treatment room when he did pelvic tilt exercises.

It's usually easy while sitting to get someone to rock his or her pelvis forward. We just say, "Sit up as tall as you can" and just like that, the pelvis will rock forward.

As easy as it is to do this in a sitting position, it can be very awkward for some people when lying down. We don't have gravity to work against. We don't have our height measured lying down, so being asked to lengthen the spine in bed or on the floor isn't familiar. But doing pelvic rocking and spinal lengthening while lying down is a great way to work on the coordination of the muscles that move and stabilize the spine and to get them out of spasm.

Slumping is easy to do when we're sitting because we're letting gravity have its way with us. If we're sitting on a stool and using no effort to sit erect, we'll end up slumping. The back rounds out and the chin juts out if we want to look forward. When we're lying on our side, we have to work at slumping. We have to use muscles to get the back to round out as far as it can. This is a good thing, as it stretches back muscles while we're using abdominal muscles. If the back is strained and in spasm, we'll feel the pull as it rounds out. Then we'll realize, "Oh, that's where my back is strained," if we didn't know already.

Getting Out of Bed

It's not so much "getting out of the wrong side of the bed" as getting out of the bed wrong.

- If lying on the back, bend knees so feet are flat on the bed.
- Roll to the side, keeping hips and shoulders in line. Don't twist shoulders forward without having hips follow shoulders.
- Now, lying on the side, push up with arms and let legs move off the edge of the bed into a sitting position.
- Scoot forward to the edge of bed with feet on floor.
- Straighten up into PIL position and stand up.

Getting Into Bed

- Sit on the edge of the bed.
- Lie on side and lift legs up onto bed.
- Roll onto back with feet flat and knees bent.

SLUMP/PIL IN SIDE-LYING

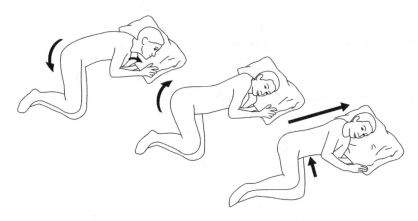

• Start with rocking the pelvis backward, rounding out the back.
• Then rock the pelvis forward, arching or straightening the back.
• Repeat back and forth a few times.
• With the pelvis rocked backward and the back rounded out, add jutting the chin forward. This is a slump position in side-lying.
• Now, rock the pelvis forward and lengthen the spine. Take time to do this. The head and the upper back will have to move backward on the bed and pillow to fully straighten and lengthen the spine.
• Tuck in the chin, lengthening the back of the neck.
• Pull the belly in towards the spine and pinch the shoulder blades slightly together and down.
• Check the lengthening of the spine and back of the neck, keeping the shoulders down. Check that the teeth are apart and the tongue is resting on the roof of the mouth.
• Take a few deep breaths holding the PIL position.
• Relax and repeat a few times. Then roll on the other side and repeat.

Note: We can also do PIL when we're lying on the back with or without a pillow under our head. If lying with legs out straight is uncomfortable, bend knees so that feet are flat on the bed.

If lying down is uncomfortable, use towels and pillows for support in bed to be more comfortable before doing these exercises (pp. 101 and 102).

Acute Spinal Strain

For an acute strain from trauma—heavy lifting injury, car accident—start by pulling the belly in towards the spine without any pelvic movement. After a more severe injury or flare-up, it's good to take short walks, avoid too much sitting, and focus on pulling the belly in with the spine comfortably lengthened. It's best not to do too much pelvic wiggling around those first few days. Use ice for 1-3 days (15-20 minutes, 3-4 times a day) and then switch to heat (10-15 minutes), doing these gentle exercises and then use ice again, if needed (p. 103). After 1-3 days we can start trying these Slump/PIL movements slowly.

If it feels too painful, then continue pulling in the belly with the spine lengthened and wait until later or the next day to try these movements again. It's very important to get the spine moving slowly in an anti-gravity position—in bed or on the floor, side-lying or on hands and knees. For faster recovery of a back strain, focus on keeping the spine erect and frequently pulling in the belly (PIL) when upright.

Note: You can always try to do these exercises after an acute injury and see how they feel. You're not going to hurt yourself worse by lying on your side and moving slowly, stopping where pain increases. It may be easier to begin in the hands and knees position (cat-camel) for slow spinal and pelvic movements (p. 130). This is often easier to begin with than Slump/PIL.

When to Seek Medical Attention for Spinal Pain

- Changes in bowel and/or bladder function, resulting in incontinence or difficulty controlling bowel movements, or numbness around the anus or genital region.
- Muscle weakness in your arms or legs, not due to pain. This is an inability to lift your foot or grip with your hand.
- Pain and numbness that travels down both arms and/or legs, especially if sneezing, coughing, or sitting down makes it worse.
- Pain that worsens when you're lying down or that keeps you awake at night.
- Pain accompanied by fever, weight loss, or other signs of illness.

Reminder

If it's too uncomfortable to do PIL in standing, try doing Slump/ PIL in sitting. If doing PIL in sitting is too uncomfortable, do Slump/PIL lying down.

After doing PIL in sitting, stand up, keeping the back straight. Try slowly arching backward with hands supporting the back. Do PIL again in standing and start walking slowly, keeping a lengthened spine. Maybe it's just a short walk at first.

If things are bad enough, apply some ice or heat to the back for 10 to 15 minutes and try doing it again. Doing PIL while sitting or lying down with heat on the back or neck is good, too (p. 103).

SUMMARY OF PART TWO

1. Using PIL (Postural Isometric Lengthening) gives immediate relief from spinal pain. Lengthening and strengthening the spine can be done while sitting, standing, walking, or lying in bed.

2. Spinal symptoms can include neck, mid, and low back aches and pains. In addition, pain, numbness, tingling, or aching into the arms or legs may come from the spine—known as referred pain.

3. PIL is also the first thing to do if having pain in the jaw, shoulder, or hip as all of these joints have muscular attachments to the spine.

4. Making a habit of doing PIL during the day makes us more aware of ourselves in the moment and is stress relieving. Doing PIL frequently can both treat spinal strains and prevent us from having them.

5. PIL is especially good to do when we're driving or sitting for long distance traveling, or when doing any prolonged sitting. We usually need to scoot hips back deeper into the seat to do PIL as the bottom slides forward as we sit.

6. Slump/PIL is especially good to do in bed before sleeping and after waking.

PART THREE

Chapter 7

Might Need a Tune Up
Body Mechanics

*A**man in his late 50s attended our Friday afternoon Back Class. His back pain was so severe he couldn't stand up straight. He'd injured himself while packing up his apartment, and had to move out and into a new place that weekend. He couldn't really participate in the class, but paid careful attention to all the do's and don'ts about lifting and bending.*

I scheduled him for an individual appointment with me the next week, assuming he was going to need more help than just the class. He arrived, walking with a spritely step and said he felt so good that he could have cancelled his appointment but just wanted to make sure he was OK. I asked what miracle occurred since I'd seen him last. He said it was moving out of his apartment carrying boxes up and down stairs, loading and unloading the truck using "perfect" body mechanics! It was painful at first, but as he warmed up and got stronger he felt great. Not the usual PT prescription, "Go load and unload heavy boxes, walk up and down stairs, until your pain goes away." But it did work.

Some people have a hard time making the connection between why they hurt and what they did to make themselves hurt. More people are unaware of what they do that's continuing to make them hurt. "Good" body mechanics and postural habits make you stronger and more flexible. "Bad" ones cause more strain to joints, weaken muscles and make sensory nerves more sensitive—setting you up for chronic pain conditions.

Awareness of body mechanics (how we move) and postural habits (moving in and out of static positions, taking breaks, walking) is the key to both avoiding injury and to pain relief.

The good news is that good body mechanics are really quite simple. The only tricky part is that they need to be applied to some awkward situations that life throws our way. Think of PIL—especially with standing and walking—as a safety net if strains happen.

Lifting and working "wrong" basically means bending and twisting the spine as we lift and work. If our shoulders are going in one direction and the pelvis is going in another, we're twisting the spine. An easy way to know we're not twisting the spine is that the belly button is between the hands when we work, lift, or sit in a chair. Then shoulders and pelvis are lined up right. If hands are both to one side and the belly is facing the other way, we're twisting the spine.

When we reach down sideways to hoist something up with one hand, that's side-bending—which also twists the spine. Twisting and side-bending when working or lifting weight, is not using good body mechanics.

Becoming aware of something we do many times a day, such as lifting ourselves out of a chair, is a good way to begin perfecting good body mechanics.

Delaying Recovery—Too Much Stretching

Often bending forward is painful with a back strain. Pain with bending forward will improve with time, but we can't start off trying to bend to get better. Soon after an injury, bending and twisting the spine against gravity—while standing or sitting—needs to be avoided in order to recover. Many people think that they just need to stretch out some problem in their back and do forward bending stretching during the day. This is a big mistake. By only doing forward bending stretches—like knee to chest exercises—muscles that are strained from being stretched too much, are getting stretched even more. Over-stretching greatly delays recovery and can cause chronic pain condition—when these strained muscles really need to be strengthened.

We can avoid additional strain to the back, and promote healing and strengthening, by using good body mechanics that bend ankles, knees, and hips and keep the back straight.

STANDING UP AND SITTING DOWN

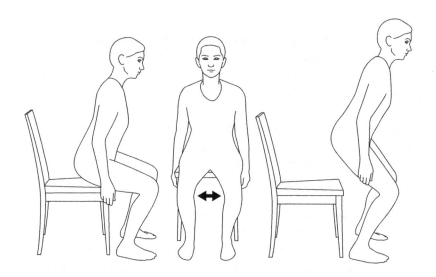

- Scoot to the edge of the chair.
- Start with sitting tall before standing.
- Feet parallel—or close to parallel—about shoulder width apart or less.
- Knees open, bending over feet, or exaggerate and have knees open wider than feet, like riding a horse.
- Look ahead and keep back erect, chest open.
- Bend forward in hips.
- Stand up using legs, keeping back straight—"hinging" at hips, looking forward.
- Sit down with feet parallel, about shoulder width apart.
- Keep head up, looking forward, with back straight. Hinging at hips, sit down slowly in chair, bending knees over feet. Or exaggerate and have knees open wider than feet. Don't flop or fall into a chair.

If we can't get out of a chair without using arms and pushing up, an easy way to strengthen the hips and legs is to practice standing up from a higher seat. We'll need some exercise equipment for this one. But fortunately it's just having a firm chair—not one with a squishy seat—placed against a wall or anything else that won't move.

CHAIR SQUATS

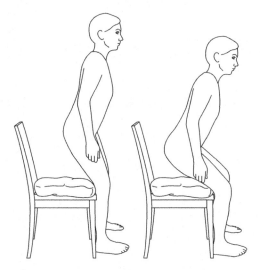

- Have a chair with a firm seat placed against a wall, preferably with armrests to hold the pillows and folded towels stacked in the seat. Make the seat the lowest height that you can stand up from without using hands.
- Stand in front of the chair with the back of legs touching the edge of the chair seat.
- Feet parallel. Bend the knees slightly wider than the feet (bow legged).
- Keep the head looking forward. Slowly sit deep into the chair, keeping the back of the legs in contact with the chair.
- To do repetitions, don't relax in the chair, but immediately stand up again slowly, keeping feet parallel, knees open wide, head up and back straight, bending in hips.
- Repeat sitting down and standing up. After we're able to do this 10 times, remove a folded towel or small pillow and continue to work on this using the lower seat height. Continue to progress by removing pillows and towels until this can be done from a regular seat height.
- If done diligently, at least 3-5 times daily or as often as every hour, many people can stand up from a regular chair without using their hands in 1-2 weeks.

LIFTING SOMETHING OFF THE FLOOR

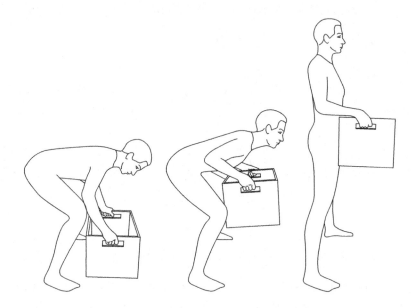

- Get close to the object you're about to lift. If something is in the way, move it aside.
- Face what you're lifting and and spread feet wide. To avoid twisting, whatever the hands are doing, the belly needs to be between the hands.
- Bend knees slightly and bend forward in the hips keeping back straight. Get a good grip on what's being lifted. While still bent forward, lift object towards belly. Elbows should be close to the waist at this point.
- Look forward—not at ground—as you stand up. This keeps the back straight. The more awkward or heavy a lift, the better to exaggerate having the head up and feet spread wide—even look up towards the ceiling.
- Stand up by straightening hips and knees.

Note: If unable to lift object by just using arms, it's too heavy. Get help or make the load lighter.

If arms are extended when lifting, it's a big strain on the back. For instance, reaching over something to grab a grocery bag off the floor, or a suitcase off the conveyor belt. In this case you have some choices:

> **1. Get closer to the item being lifted;**
> **2. Move something out of the way;**
> **3. Pull it closer before lifting.**

It Hurts, But It Hurts Good

Already injured? Often getting up from a chair is one of the most uncomfortable things to do when the back is hurting. Being careful with how we stand up is an important step to healing any acute back injury. We especially need to use the legs more to avoid further strain to the back. We often need to have feet spread wider than usual. Even though it may feel difficult and painful to do, being very aware of standing up and sitting down with the spine erect—feet and knees spread wide and head up—will help to strengthen the back and legs. This hastens recovery. It's also a very good idea to avoid any low seats when the back is injured. Try adding some cushions to make a low seat higher.

Perfect Practice

It's not just "practice that makes perfect." It's "perfect practice" that makes perfect. As we consistently repeat an activity perfectly, our neural circuitry is recording that movement. Our brains have the quality of plasticity, which means new memories of movement can be made. By using good body mechanics consistently they become new "muscle memories" and habits, replacing old memories and poor body mechanics. Whenever we notice that we haven't stood up from a chair or lifted something light using good mechanics, repeat the movement correctly. The "straw that broke the camel's back" is a common saying for a common way of injuring the back, not with a heavy lift but with the cumulative effect of many casual, awkward movements.

LIFTING SOMETHING OVERHEAD

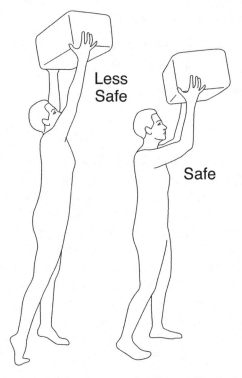

Common sense goes a long way with lifting safely. Lifting something overhead can also be risky. Many of us have seen people struggling to get their heavy luggage into the overhead compartment of planes — or have been that person. The overhead lift can make us arch the back too much under weight. It's the opposite way of hurting ourselves than with a bending lift, but we hurt ourselves just the same. The solution is to avoid arching backward by keeping the stomach pulled in. If the bag is very heavy and we're not very strong, we need help. Usually there's someone around who is happy to lend a hand.

And if we're at home and trying to get the heavy box of seasonal decorations back on the top shelf of the closet, and maybe we're standing on a wobbly stool, what are the options? Get a more stable chair or stepladder. Get some of the weight out of that box and have two lighter boxes. Get a bigger, stronger someone to do it for us! Common sense.

GOLFER'S LIFT

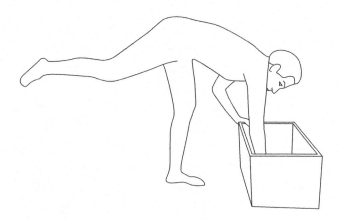

- Additional lifting technique for light lifting is known as the "golfer's lift." If lifting something light, like a piece of clothing off the floor, reach forward with one hand on a nearby object for balance.
- Slightly bend the knee on the standing leg and lift opposite leg backward keeping spine straight.
- Tilt forward and lift with the free hand.

Once something is being carried, get the shoulder blades pressed down and together—like with PIL. This helps strengthen the deep muscles of the shoulders that stabilize the shoulder joints. Make that extra effort to pull in the belly as we carry what we've lifted. Doing this while working strengthens the body's deep stabilizing muscles. Carrying the groceries into the house, taking out the garbage, schlepping around suitcases when traveling—can become a total body workout without going to the gym!

When standing from a low seat or lifting something from the floor, get feet wider than usual before standing, and straighten the back. Don't look at the floor when standing up. The heavier or more awkward the lift, look up towards the ceiling.

PULLING

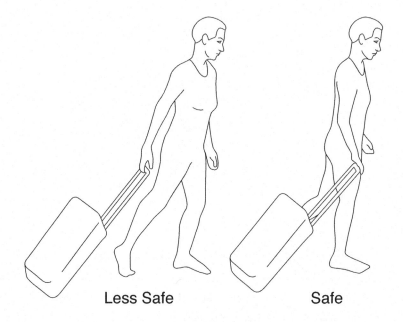

Less Safe   Safe

Another great way—on a not so great list— to hurt the back is by pulling something that's too heavy, especially if it's stuck and we try to jerk it lose. Feet are planted and we're twisting the spine as the arm pulls to one side. The spine is twisted when the shoulders are facing one way and the pelvis is facing another.

A very common pulling scenario is when traveling and hauling luggage all over the airport and through the parking lot over bumpy surfaces. The key is keeping the shoulders and hips facing forward as we walk. Also keep the elbow close to the waist as we pull the luggage. In other words, don't have the arm that's pulling the suitcase—or anything we're pulling with one arm—way behind us. If the working arm is behind, it will strain the shoulder and twist the spine.

PUSHING

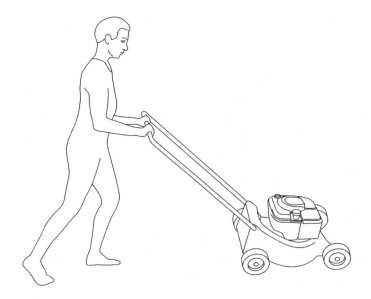

Much better, when we have a choice, is to be pushing something instead of pulling it. Pushing a weight makes it much easier to keep the back still, with elbows close to the waist, shoulder blades pulled together and down, and belly tightened. If it's a heavy load, we can move the legs while everything else is in a safe, stable position. Pushing is also an excellent isometric strengthening workout. Think of using a wheelbarrow up a slight hill or pushing a heavy shopping cart to the car. We really can feel the abdominal muscles working as well as the hips and thighs.

Back Pain with Standing

Standing on hard surfaces, like a concrete floor, can often be very uncomfortable and the back, legs, hips, knees, ankle, and feet begin to ache. The best solution is to get a foam pad to stand on at work areas, or to get foam shoes or shoe inserts to decrease the impact of hard surfaces throughout the lower body.

WORK AND PLAY: DAILY ACTIVITIES

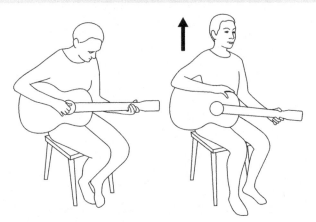

Often, when working or playing, we can get away with being in the not-so-perfect position, and we're OK. Then we might strain ourselves doing something else and when we go back to work or sit at the computer, we've become quite miserable.

Maybe we didn't notice how we were sitting on the edge of the bed and twisted as we folded clothes. Or we were bent forward as we were cooking, never straightening up at all for an hour, and by the time we sit down to eat, the back is killing us. Or we're using a vacuum and suddenly we notice that we're only thinking about "I can't wait to lie down." Then we might notice that we've just been standing in one spot twisting as we pushed and pulled the vacuum in all directions around us, frantically trying to get the job done faster. Often we hurt ourselves when we're in a hurry and throw caution and good body mechanics to the wind.

Note: Good body mechanics do not slow us down. Bad body mechanics— twisting and bending the spine with lifting/pushing/pulling— slow our whole lives down as we recover from injury.

Whenever we feel strain while working, standing, or sitting, take a second to do PIL. Then we can see how far forward we're bent or how much we've been twisting. Often we think we're standing up straight as we're doing something, but with the head looking down at what's being worked on, the back follows.

Sometimes we need to take more breaks. Short walks are good. Or take a moment to sit down and do PIL. We can stand erect occasionally as we're working—like when folding clothes, washing dishes, or brushing teeth. Stand up straight occasionally while doing any of these things. So simple, but like everything, we have to notice what we're doing first. Then it will become easy.

Working intensely on projects like painting or sculpture, playing music, pottery making, woodworking, or using power tools, often means we need to be in some awkward positions. Certainly we don't want to be thinking about postural stuff when it's much more important to be thinking, "Keep sharp blades away from fingers." But there's the work-and-play time and then there's the in-between-work-and-play time. When we're working/playing/creating, we're intent on what the hands are doing. Usually, eyes need to be on the project, and maybe the head is forward and back is bent more than ideal. Then there's the in-between time when we're walking over to get another piece of wood, or more clay or paint, or we're between songs. This is when doing PIL and hand, elbow, and shoulder exercises (Chapter 13) is a great idea.

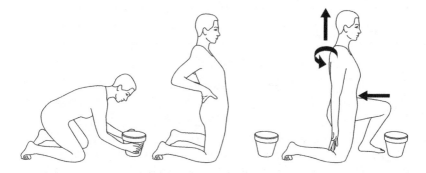

Gardening and plumbing—like working under a sink—offer different challenges. We're often tempted to sit on the floor or ground, or squat, because that's where we're working. And we can do this briefly, but we need to stand, straighten up into a kneeling position, or change to hands and knee positions, to give the back a break. Working on hands and knees is often a better option in these circumstances. Use kneepads or a kneeling pad to protect the knees. Working in a half-kneeling position or lying on the side is the better option. But no matter what, squatting down, or sitting on the ground while using both hands reaching forward for any length of time, is hard on the back.

Best advice with awkward work positions:
- *Untangle ourselves after we've been in goofy positions for too long.*
- *Get in a half kneeling position or stand up, do PIL and then arch backwards slightly.*
- *Don't go back to doing forward bending work until we're able to arch backwards comfortably.*

Best advice for standing up from sitting on floor:
- *Turn sideways, onto hands and knees.*
- *Push with arms, getting feet on the ground, feet spread wide.*
- *Walk hands towards legs and get one hand at a time on thighs above knees.*
- *With hands above bent knees, look forward.*
- *Push with arms and stand up, straightening knees and hips, keeping back straight.*

Be Good to the Knees

"Housemaid's knees" is prepatellar bursitis—inflamed bursa, sensitive soft tissue in front of the kneecap (p. 112). Sadly, a housemaid down on the hard floor scrubbing away, day in and day out, is just the kind of work that causes this problem. To avoid it, wear kneepads or use a cushioned kneeling pad when working on knees.

REPETITIVE ACTIVITIES

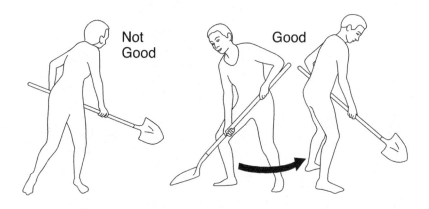

Doing repetitive activities requires some thought and planning to make sure we avoid injury. We might be shoveling from a pile of compost in front of us into the wheelbarrow behind us, or moving a pile of bricks from one place to another. It's key to pick up the feet to keep the shoulders and pelvis in line with each other, and keep the belly between the hands. This is true of weed eating and vacuuming as well. "Planting" the feet and twisting in different directions is certain to strain the back. If you can't easily pivot on the feet—often the case if needing a cane to walk due to weakness or balance problems (Chapter 8)—you can't safely be doing these activities that require pivoting.

The same idea applies to sports. Sports are high-level, often repetitive activities. An effective warm-up for any sport can be to practice good form slowly and perfectly, and then gradually increase the speed. When doing any one-side-dominant sport it's also good to warm up and cool down by moving in the non-dominant direction. For instance, if you throw right-handed, slowly do the movement of throwing left-handed.

WORKING WITH COMPUTERS

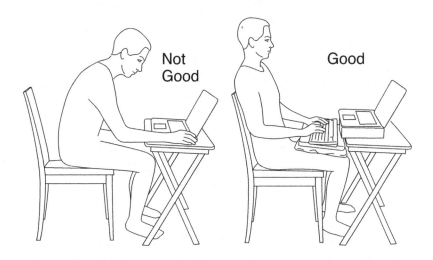

No matter how great our ergonomic set up is, we'll most likely start slumping at a computer before too long. We want to set up our workspace as well as we can, but we still need to do PIL and Slump/PIL occasionally if we're at a computer for any length of time.

When using computers, as with any work we focus on, vision rules and posture will follow. If a screen is too high, we'll jut the chin forward so we can see it. If a screen is too low, we'll slump down in the seat and then jut the chin forward to look at it. If we have a very fancy computer chair that reclines and has head support, then we can recline in a good position for working at a computer. But those of us who don't have a deluxe computer chair can still create a safe, well-designed workspace.

Our eyes are pretty comfortable looking down at about a 20-degree angle. What this translates into is that if we're sitting up nice and straight, eyes looking straight ahead should be at the top of the screen. Then our eyes can comfortably gaze downward (approximately 20 degrees from the horizontal), to look at the screen below. Check this while doing PIL.

With a laptop, the screen can be pushed back to have eyes gaze downward comfortably. With a monitor we might have to make some adjustments to get this right. We can raise the monitor simply by putting something under it, like books we don't intend to look at ever again. Make sure it's one of our own books—"Honey, have you seen that book I was reading?" Or we can raise the height of the chair.

When using a keyboard or a mouse, keep elbows near the waist and wrists fairly straight. Reaching forward or outward to use a mouse can be the reason for having a problem with the wrist, elbow, shoulder, neck, or a referred nerve pain from the neck. You can complain to human resources, but unless they're really quick in coming to the rescue, we're our own best human resource.

This isn't to say we shouldn't report our ergonomic problems at work. But it's good to work on our own temporary solutions until they can get us fixed up. And if we're working for ourselves as independents, or temp contractors, or we just like to spend an inordinate amount of time at our laptops or home computers, then we have to figure out our own solutions.

If we're sitting at an old-style office desk without any accommodations for computers, open the upper side drawer and place a book over the drawer. Voila! Here's a place for the mouse to go. If the keyboard is sitting on a desk too high for wrists to be straight, put the keyboard on top of a big firm pillow on the lap. A keyboard or mouse can be plugged into a laptop if needed. Be creative!

Sometimes the whole computer isn't directly in front of us. We're slightly twisted when using the computer and then twisting the other direction to reach for a phone or files. We can fix this by rearranging the desk until we are sitting right in front of the keyboard and computer screen. The basic swivel chair lets us shift our pelvis around to face whatever we might be reaching for, including that lower desk drawer. If we don't have that swivel chair, we need to lift ourselves up and shift the pelvis—use the legs—so the belly is facing what we're doing with the hands. Remember, side bending is twisting, too!

These are the funky workstations of life that we'll often have to work with if we don't have the perfect workspace. Take more breaks doing PIL, and do the shoulder and hand stretches (Chapter 13). Throw in a little neural mobilization (Chapter 15) for good measure! We could get a relatively inexpensive adjustable computer workstation to alternate between sitting and standing. If we sit a lot in our lives, we need to balance that out by taking walks. This is a good idea for lots of reasons—it improves circulation, it's good for muscles, joints, nerves, and general well being. Bodies need to move.

Note: Important to remember that the body is more like those of hunter-gatherers and less like computer automatons. Technology has changed. Our bodies haven't.

SMARTPHONES

Why do smartphones make us do foolish things? And it's not just being distracted while walking into oncoming traffic, or getting into an accident while driving and using one. By now we should be able to look at anyone using a smartphone and figure out why they're rubbing their neck. The key to avoiding smartphone injuries is to hold the phone up so the spine can be straight. Take frequent breaks to fully straighten up. Yes, PIL again. And then, let go of it every now and then to stretch out hands and fingers wide like signaling a distant waiter for a table for five with the elbow straight. Especially stretch wide between the thumb and index finger (p. 164). Using smartphones is a really foolish way to get hurt.

Tips for Low Back Pain on One Side

Good tips for one sided back pain: Try to keep the hip on the painful side straight when working. That means, if we're in a half kneeing position, have the painful side's knee on the ground—that hip is then straight. If we're doing a golfer's lift, swing back the leg on the sore side to keep that hip straight. If we need to step up on a high step, use the leg on the side that isn't sore. Avoid anything that brings the sore side's knee in closer to the chest.

Tips for Bending and Reaching

When reaching with the arm extended, it's best to have some forward support to avoid excessive strain on the back. If there's nothing around to lean on—like when reaching deep in the refrigerator or into a low drawer—we can lean on ourselves. Feet spread wide, elbow on knee for reaching downward; hand on knee for reaching forward.

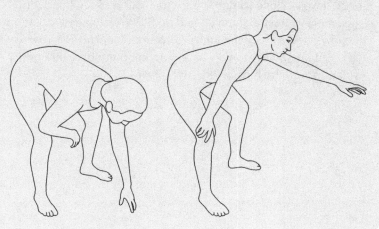

A Quick Fix

If we can't be in these good positions when lifting, pushing, or pulling, we need to get help. It's really not worth it to injure the back and have it hurting for weeks. But, if we do something that we wish we hadn't, as soon as we can, stand up straight, do PIL and then slowly, with hands supporting the low back, arch backwards. It's a quick fix for a moment's indiscretion. If we can't stand up straight we need to find a place to sit down and do PIL while sitting at the edge of the seat.

It's a very good idea not to do any more bending until arching backwards feels good. Be especially careful with how we sit when driving and relax at home after a strain. Good to do PIL frequently and to do Slump/PIL in sidelying (p. 57) or cat-camel on hands and knees (p. 130) when we can.

Reminder

It's worth repeating: For a healthy, happy back we should always be able to stand up straight and arch backward. We can bend with a straight back, but we can't stand straight with a bent back. If we've done something to strain our backs, we should immediately try to straighten up and do PIL. With hands supporting the low back, arch back slightly. Once that's feeling OK, then we can continue by being very careful to keep the back straight as we bend with the hips, knees, and ankles.

Chapter 8

Take It In Stride
Balance and Walking

In the same way that lifting with poor body mechanics can cause injury or delay recovery, walking with a limp can have the same effect. Of course some people have few options of how to walk due to major injuries, surgeries (limited joint mobility) or neurologic conditions (limited strength or coordination). Without these kinds of limitations, trying to protect a healed injury that's still painful by walking awkwardly can lead to more complicated problems. Walking slowly with a normal gait is literally the first step to recovery.

We already know that walking slowly doing PIL can relieve back pain. Though we've been doing it all our lives, once we're able to resume walking after having an injury or surgery involving the legs, we often forget exactly how we used to walk. We might start walking with a stiff knee or take a step with a flat foot. By walking "normally"—though slower and with a shorter step—our mobility and strength begins to improve naturally. Take the time to read below and then walk, being conscious of what feet, ankles, and knees are doing. Being barefoot or wearing flexible shoes will make this easier to do.

WALKING BASICS

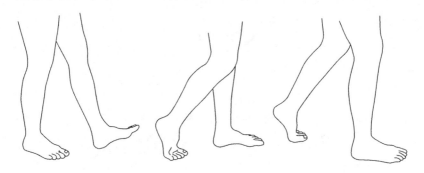

- Begin by doing PIL while standing.
- Take a step forward. The heel hits the ground first. The knee is slightly bent.

Note: With ankle injuries, we often step onto a flat foot. Heel strike helps with ankle mobility and strengthening.

- Continue to move forward. Full weight is on the foot, with weight on the outer border and all toes in contact with the ground. Knee is still slightly bent.

Note: Having all our weight on a locked, or fully straightened knee, prevents us from using the quadriceps—muscles in the front of the thigh. A slightly bent knee is key to getting that muscle working well again. Encouraging an active arch in the foot is good to prevent foot injuries and keep the foot strong.

- Swing through with other leg by bending the knee and straightening it ahead.
- Moving forward from the foot we're standing on, push off the BIG toe.

Note: Walking and rolling over the arch and the side of the big toe (knocked kneed walking) weakens and stiffens the big toe and strains the arch. This can lead to getting bunions and plantar fasciitis.

- The heel strikes on the other leg with knee slightly bent as we take the next step forward.

A few more points:

- *As weight is on one leg, the hip—actually the pelvis—on that side rises up and the side with the leg swinging through drops down. This makes for a nice hip-swinging gait. Some people swing their hips more than others. Think Marilyn Monroe versus John Wayne.*
- *Doing PIL while we're walking will take some hip swing out of the gait. When the low back is sore, often this is a good idea and makes walking much easier.*
- *Head and shoulders should stay fairly still in relation to the rest of the body and not sway side to side too much. Lots of swaying is typical of hip weakness.*
- *Slow, mindful walking—being very aware of the foot position in contact with the floor and knee movement—is also great for any foot, ankle, knee, or hip pain. It's good to make the heel strike slightly on its outer border. Moving from the outer border of the foot before pushing off the big toe encourages ankle and foot rotational strength.*

What can happen, as we get older—especially if we've already had a fall—is that we start being fearful of falling again and we begin to look down as we walk. Wearing bifocal glasses or progressive lenses makes looking at the floor fuzzy and then we want to bend even more to see the floor. Looking at the ground—because we feel our balance is off—actually makes our balance worse. With the head bent forward, balance sensors in our inner ears that work with our vision, can't recognize this new orientation to the world. We're not getting the same message to the brain about the body being upright. Adding insult to injury, necks and backs become strained and painful as we walk bent forward looking down.

This is when we need to practice PIL in a sitting position at the edge of a seat, looking forward to get the head and body used to that upright position again. PIL helps strengthen trunk muscles by pulling in the belly and holding that lengthened posture, having the head aligned over the body.

Then, in a standing position, practice PIL. Hold onto something at first for balance. Getting used to being upright while doing PIL helps with strength and balance. If we can't stand up from a chair without using arms we need to practice the chair squat strengthening (p. 67).

Note: Avoid having clutter on the floor. Take up any small slippery rugs that could cause a fall. Be careful with small pets and their toys. Have rooms well lit with nightlights. Have a flashlight by the bedside if power goes out.

STANDING BALANCE

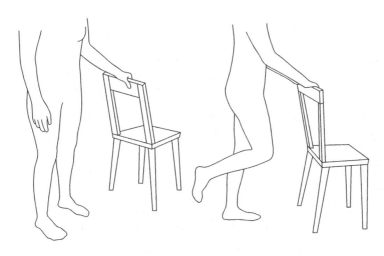

- Stand facing the kitchen counter, hands on the counter and do PIL. Stand with feet shoulder width for 10 seconds.
- Then, without swaying or wobbling, slowly lift up one hand. If that goes OK, then lift up the other hand. Stand for 10 seconds. The body makes balance adjustments to keep us standing there.
- To make it more challenging, stand with feet together for 10 seconds.
- Turn and stand sideways to the counter. Now just one hand is touching the counter for balance. Again, stand with feet close together while doing PIL, and try to keep standing up straight without wobbling around. Then try lifting the hand off the counter. Keep the hand near the counter, in case we need to use it.
- Facing the kitchen counter, try standing on one leg with fingertips on the counter, keeping the pelvis level—no side bending—while doing PIL. Try to maintain balance with the knee slightly bent, lifting one hand and then both hands.
- Normal balance is maintaining balance on one leg, without using fingertips for support, for 10 seconds.

FORWARD AND SIDEWAYS WALKING

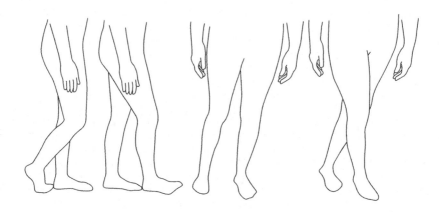

- We can improve our gait by walking slowly forward and backward while having a hand on the kitchen counter or back of a couch.
- To make it more challenging, walk heel to toe.
- Face the counter and take steps sideways, keeping head up and back straight, touching the counter, or whatever is available for balance.
- To make it more challenging, cross one leg over the other walking sideways.

HELP WITH WALKING

If we're not able to walk well—if we're recovering from injury, having problems with balance or unable to keep the trunk erect for one reason or another—we need to use something to help stability. It doesn't necessarily have to be forever if we work to improve our strength and balance with walking and sit to stand. But when we can't balance at all on either leg for a few seconds, then we need to have a cane, walking stick, or a crutch. If both legs are a problem we might need two canes, two walking poles, two crutches, or a walker. If we really can't walk, we need a wheelchair.

Plenty of people whom I'd see in the clinic weren't too happy about this prospect. "I don't want to use that. That will make me look old."

If I could get away with it, I'd say, "So you think you look good the way you're walking now?"

The purpose of using any assistive walking device is to make walking normal and safer. If we're just having problems with one leg or one side, then we can try using a cane. Although counterintuitive, use the cane on the side opposite of the weaker leg. It's the same if we're using one crutch or walking pole. Use it on the opposite side as we step on the weaker leg. Having it opposite of the injured leg or back creates the effect of standing on two feet. If we use it on the weaker side, we lean sideways into it, side-bending the back in the process. That being said, I've certainly seen people who just couldn't use the cane the "proper" way. Try it on the opposite side. If it just doesn't work, try not to bend sideways using it in the not-proper way. Once again, doing PIL occasionally while walking will help avoid side-bending.

Ideally, if we need to use crutches or a walker, we're being fitted and shown how to use them by a health professional. Since that isn't always the case, here are some of the main points.

ADJUSTING CRUTCHES, CANES, AND WALKERS

Adjust the height of canes, crutches, and walkers while standing in an erect posture.

Crutches need to be adjusted to allow two inches between the top of the crutch and the armpit. The length of the crutch and the level of the handgrip can both be adjusted. If we lean on them, arms can start to get numb as the nerves and blood vessels in the arm pit are getting cut off from blood supply. As we push down on the handgrips, elbows should be slightly bent.

A cane should be adjusted so the elbow is slightly bent when the cane is at the side. Shoulders should be down and not shrugged up.

Walkers should also be adjusted so the elbows slightly bend and are at the side while standing. Just like with a cane or crutch, elbows should be slightly bent and close to the side when walking with a walker. Avoid pushing the walker ahead by bending forward with arms out straight and elbows away from the body.

We should be able to walk well with any of these devices. That means standing up erect, occasionally doing PIL, head over the body, and eyes looking forward. Walk slowly until getting the hang of it. Just because we have something to help us walk doesn't mean we should go speeding off.

If we're having trouble with balance or we're falling, it's really important to let people know—family, friends, doctors. That being said, it's very common not to tell anyone when we've had a fall or are fearful of falling. The fear is not just about falling. It's fear of the end of independence and mobility. It's admitting that "I'm getting old," and so many of us want nothing to do with that.

We first need to notice changes with walking and balance, and then we can do something about it. Falls can be a game changer. We think that we're hiding the fact that we're not walking well by not using a cane or walker. But anyone can see when we're having trouble with balance. It's a common problem. Better to face it and get help than to stop moving and become less active and weaker for fear of falling. "Facing it" means being honest with yourself and being mindful of getting stronger and improving balance by including the balance practice (pp. 87 and 88) and chair squat strengthening (p. 67) in our daily lives. Or see a physical therapist for help. In the meantime, continue to walk safely with a cane or walker.

Reminder

As we become older, some of us walk beautifully. For others, maybe we don't walk so well. Even if we used to walk well, whether we're older or not, balance and gait can change. It can happen fairly quickly after having spent a significant amount of time in bed (after intensive medical treatment or recovering from surgery)—or can change slowly overtime through inattention and a gradual decrease in activity. In either case, use balance exercise to test balance ability. If they're difficult to do, use these exercises—and practice slow walking while doing PIL—as a way to improve.

Chapter 9

Too Soft, Too Hard, Just Right
Chairs and Beds

I once saw a young man in his early 20s with his first onset of low
back pain. He was off from work, thinking pain pills would do
the trick to get him better, but after a couple of weeks it was evident
that the pills weren't working. He had no idea what he was supposed
to be doing for himself and got referred to physical therapy. Sitting
and bending was especially painful for him. Besides wondering if
he'd be able to get back to doing construction work, he worried that
his previously comfortable chair would never feel comfortable again.
He tried sitting in his friend's recliner chair. That was the only place
he felt comfortable. At least while he was in it. It was hellish getting up from it, but that didn't concern him as much. He thought a
recliner was what he needed, so he went out and ordered one.

The rest of his life with chronic back pain flashed before my eyes.
After hearing more of his story and doing my evaluation, I explained that resting wasn't the solution to a back pain problem and
that he would recover with some instruction about body mechanics

and strengthening. I ever so tactfully recommended that he cancel his recliner chair order.

When spines—neck, mid back, and low back—are strained (muscle injury), sprained (ligament or disc injury), or recovering from surgery, they are weakened and become less stable. Chairs, car seats, and beds that had felt comfortable often become intolerable. We need to rely on more support from chairs and beds to be able to relax comfortably, to allow sprained ligaments and discs to heal, and to avoid having muscles go into spasm.

To better understand taking care of a back injury, it's often easier to picture a sprained ankle. After an ankle has been twisted we wrap it firmly in a straight alignment in order for it to heal.

Spraining the low back and then sitting in a soft chair that rounds the back out is just like keeping that sprained ankle in a twisted inward position—the position of the injury. Pain pills, usually given or offered after a traumatic injury or flare up of neck and back pain, make us less aware of pain as we sit without added support. These pills help with the pain but also inadvertently help us tolerate sitting without support. But we shouldn't be fooled! Taking pain pills makes us less aware of pain, but also less aware of the effects of a non-supportive chair or bed on an injury. Added support to chairs is an essential part of good early self-care for any spine injury, recovery from surgery, or flare-up.

IMPROVING CHAIRS

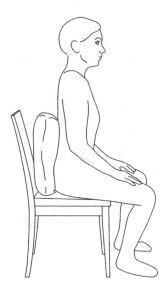

We can always perch on the edge of a chair and fairly easily maintain an erect posture. But this gets tiring and we want to be able to relax and rest the back against something.

- Find a firm level seat that's easy to do PIL in. OK to add a pillow on the seat for comfort. Wooden chairs, kitchen or dining room chairs often are the best. Avoid using seats that tilt the pelvis backwards—like a bucket seat or worn out upholstered chair— or that tilt the pelvis sideways—one hip higher than the other.
- If a bucket seat or soft furniture can't be avoided, place a folded towel or a small blanket in the back half of the seat, towards the backrest. Buttocks are on the blanket/towel, thighs on the seat.
- If the seat is tilted sideways, we need more height on the lower side.
- Sitting on a level seat, scoot hips back deep in the seat and do PIL. (Don't forget that PIL is lengthening, not arching, the spine.) While doing PIL note how far away the back is from the seat back. That's the amount of space that needs to be filled in with a rolled or folded towel or pillow.

• With acute pain, often a small firm rolled towel is needed along
the sacrum—the lowest part of the spine—to maintain the forward position of the pelvis. Try folding a small towel or a small
pillow and place it *lengthwise* between the buttocks. Usually, now
the upper back is no longer in contact with the back of the chair.
Add a big pillow to the back of the seat to rest into.

*Note: This might take some adjusting to get the right support. Keep working
on it. An added pillow could be too big, too small, or just right. The support
might feel great at first and then becomes uncomfortable. If that's the case,
pull the support out for a few minutes and then try using it again, or adjust
the support.*

MORE TIPS ON IMPROVING CHAIRS

*Note: Another factor in finding the right pillow support for the back is the
shape of the buttocks—are they like pillows themselves, or are they spare and
boney with no curves?*

• For those of us who are well endowed, fill in a bigger space to
support the back as buttocks are against the lower part of the
backrest. Hips are scooted back deep into the seat.
• Do PIL. The back is well away from the back of the chair.
• The right pillow for the low back is often a squishy bed pillow that
will go from the lower back and up into the upper back.
• Push the pillow into the low back to give it more bulk. The rest
of the upper back can rest on the remaining pillow.
• On the other hand, those of us with flattened spines use a firm,
flat support.
• Continue to do PIL occasionally when sitting.

SITTING WITH STRUCTURAL INCREASED MID-BACK CURVE

If you have an increased forward curve in the mid-back (a structural kyphosis), sitting support has to be approached differently.

- Sitting erect, the mid-back hits the backrest before the hips reach the back of the chair. One of the best solutions is to use a squishy bed pillow.
- Sit erect and stuff the pillow between the backrest and the buttocks. Once that space is filled, use the rest of the pillow as a soft support for the mid back.
- In a recliner chair, a pillow behind the head is usually necessary to have the spine in good alignment.

Some chairs or beds are still not comfortable after adding support. If pain becomes chronic, often these chairs or beds should be avoided altogether. Getting rid of them is sometimes the best solution!

Find what's comfortable that keeps you close to a PIL position and do PIL frequently. If the back is still touchy, don't sit for too long. Be especially careful to stand up from the chair with good mechanics (p. 66). It may be painful to stand up, but being in that erect position—feet spread, knees open, head up—will help get you stronger and promote healing. If we need this much support to be comfortable, get up and take short walks while doing PIL for 1-2 minutes. Do it frequently (every 15-30 minutes) or lie down and rest occasionally.

RECLINER CHAIRS

Spines often don't like to be sitting upright all the time. We want to relax and be tilted backwards slightly. This can work if we're sitting on a couch and have some big pillows stuffed behind the back, giving more comfortable support. We still need to do PIL in reclined sitting to avoid over-stretching the back. In a car many of us need to recline the seat slightly to be comfortable.

- Recliner chairs are fine if we have problems with the circulation in the legs (swelling) and need to have them elevated.
- Recliners are also great if we have had a very severe accident, major surgery, or have a debilitating medical condition. They can make life a lot more comfortable.
- But for a basically healthy person who has focused and "catastrophized" about back pain and has become steadily less active, it's a mistake to think that recliner chairs are a solution to the problem. When a recliner chair is the only place we feel comfortable but we moan and groan as we get out of it, the trunk and legs have become weak. The spine is unstable and we need to start doing PIL like crazy! Also we need to strengthen the legs with chair squat exercise (p. 67). Be careful to use good body mechanics when standing to avoid strain to the back. Start to do more walking and moving around.

ARM SUPPORT WITH SITTING

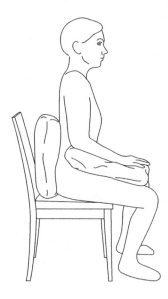

- If we're all propped up and a neck, shoulder, or arm pain is still a problem, place another pillow—or a backpack or purse—beneath the forearm. Keep the forearm parallel to the thigh.
- An adjustable armrest may need to be raised or lowered.
- Rest the elbow on the pillow or armrest. Keep it near the waist, but don't lean on it. This supports the weight of the arm.

Note: The weight of the arm without support can increase both the pain from a shoulder joint or a nerve pain coming from the neck.

SITTING ON THE FLOOR OR GROUND

Sitting on the floor or the ground is sometimes a challenge. Those of us with an older, degenerative lumbar spine—and the older body that goes with it—often avoid it. Few of us have hips flexible enough to allow the pelvis into a rocked forward position while sitting on the floor. If the spine is bent forward and pelvis rocked backward it doesn't take long to feel sore.

- If we must sit on the floor, find something to lean back on, like the base of a couch or wall, and sit on a cushion.
- If that's not an option, place arms behind and lean back on the hands. This might be tolerable for a short while.
- Occasionally rock the pelvis forward as well.

But best is to not be sitting on the floor in the first place if the back is at all touchy.

Don't Just Sit There – Do Something!

Even with all this propping up, we still want to be moving into the PIL position every so often. Remember, we're really still hunter-gatherers stuck in a modern time. The body doesn't like too much sitting, especially with an acute strain. Taking breaks to get up and walk around, standing and arching backward always help.

IMPROVING BEDS

After a severe injury to the back we often want to lie down and rest, taking short walks every hour or two. If a bed is comfortable and easy to relax into, then all is well. But if that nagging back or neck pain gets worse as soon as we're lying still, there's just no way for the shoulders to be comfortable— we have to do something about it.

LYING ON THE BACK

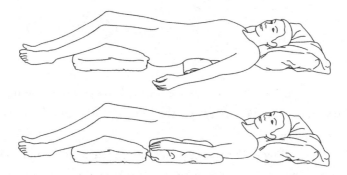

- The first thing to do is Slump/PIL (p. 57). Do it slowly in a small range of motion for an acute injury. Do it a few times lying on the side or on the back, to see if that makes things better.
- If not, the solution is once again, more pillows and towels. These props help get the spine, hips, and shoulders in positions that avoid added strain.
- Roll up or fold towels and place under the neck and back when we're lying on the back. This gives support to injured joints and strained muscles so they aren't being stretched.
- Place pillows under the knees to take strain off the back. This also helps if we have a strained knee or hip.
- If shoulders are painful, use a pillow under the elbow, not the shoulder. (With arms flat on the bed shoulders are actually stretched backward.)

LYING ON THE SIDE

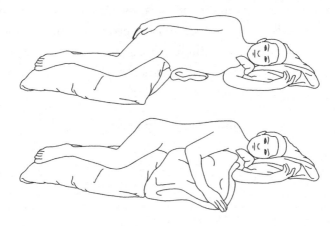

- When lying on the side, place a rolled towel under the neck or waist, and a pillow between the knees. This keeps the hips and back aligned.
- Have a pillow under the upper elbow, forearm, and hand to lessen the strain on the shoulder. Arm or leg pain coming from the spine—referred symptoms—need pillow support. Be sure to support the hand and foot.

Note: After all this propping up, we may need to do Slump/PIL in side-lying a few times to get muscles and joints more comfortable.

Lying on the Stomach

Some people like to sleep on their stomachs. Most physical therapists get uncomfortable just hearing about this. It can put the low back in an end-of-range position. To breathe, the neck is also turned to an extreme end range. Bottom line: If you wake up in the morning feeling stiff and miserable, stop sleeping on your stomach and try the other suggestions above. Or, if you start having mysterious neck and back pain, stop sleeping on your stomach and try these other suggestions. But, if after sleeping on your stomach you feel just great in the morning and your neck and back have never felt better, good for you!

Using Ice and Heat

It's very important to sit or lie with support—as described in this chapter—while using ice or heat. Otherwise we run the risk of getting more comfortable (with heat) or numb (with ice) in a strained position.

- Protect the skin with a dry cloth when using ice or heat and check the skin frequently when using either.
- Ice (packs or gel) or heat (microwavable packs, electric heating pads, hot water bottles) can be used 15-20 minutes every 2-3 hours, but not more often.
- Ice should be used with acute injuries—joint sprains, severe muscle strains and acute bursitis (p. 112)—for pain and swelling. Use for 3-7 days as needed.
- Heat can be used before doing exercises if stiffness or achy pain is a problem.
- If symptoms increase after first starting to do exercises, ice can be used again after exercise, but only if necessary.

Reminder

When we've strained the spine—neck, mid back, or low back—supportive deep muscles are not working well. That's why we need to add more support to chairs and beds—to compensate for the weakened deep muscles. We're using external support (added pillows, rolled towels, etc) to avoid putting additional strain on the weakened deep muscles and overworked superficial muscles. All this added support will not usually be necessary for comfort with sitting or lying down as we recover.

SUMMARY OF PART THREE

Chapter 7

1. Prolonged bending, twisting, stretching and prolonged slumped sitting are common ways of causing spinal pain.

2. With a flare up of spinal symptoms, prolonged bending and twisting stretches—especially if we're having referred spinal pain into the arms and legs—will make the pain worse!

3. How we stand up and sit down in a chair can keep us strong and prevent us from injuring our backs, hips, knees, ankles, and feet. Standing up with good body mechanics hastens our recovery from injury and improves our strength.

4. We can strengthen our legs by practicing chair squats slowly from a chair—making a seat higher by adding cushions and towels (p. 67).

5. Acquiring good body mechanics with lifting and all daily activities requires practicing "perfectly" with both easy and harder activities to rewire neural pathways—making good body mechanics automatic.

6. Find the short breaks in concentrative or creative work— and do PIL, arch backwards, and stretch out the hands.

7. Avoid prolonged sitting on the ground when working. Better to work on hands and knees or a half kneeling position with knee pads, or lie on the side. Only briefly squat or sit on the ground when working.

8. With any pushing, pulling, using a computer or hand held devices, belly should be facing what hands are doing, elbows should be close to sides, spine fairly erect. Do PIL as needed when working/bending/sitting.

9. Be creative by adjusting your workspace.

SUMMARY OF PART THREE

Chapter 8

1. Walking slowly with good mechanics and doing PIL can remove additional strain and promote a quicker recovery to back or leg injury.

2. With any foot, ankle, knee, or hip pain, it's very helpful to focus on how feet are in contact with the floor and to walk more slowly.

3. Our balance is affected after we've been bed ridden with illness or major injury/surgery/medical condition. Balance can be regained by practicing balance exercises and slow walking with good mechanics.

4. If we can't walk without limping, or if our balance is poor, we need to use an assistive device to prevent further injury, avoid falling, and to improve gait.

SUMMARY OF PART THREE

Chapter 9

1. Joints, muscles, and nerves need movement for health and suffer from inactivity. Stand up and take short walks. Do PIL frequently when we have to sit for longer periods.

2. Add support to seats and chairs to improve spinal alignment and pelvic position, especially with acute strains or injuries.

3. For arm pain from the neck or shoulder, support—but don't lean—on arm.

4. Firm beds are the best with varying amounts of cushioning on top. If you have to sleep on a sagging bed, add support to low back (rolled or folded towel) to help keep the spine straight.

5. Add support under knees or arms lying on back—or between legs and supporting upper arm lying on side.

6. Doing Slump/PIL in side-lying and lying on the back is good to do before going to sleep and in the morning before getting out of bed

PART FOUR

Chapter 10

The Nuts and Bolts of Movement
Anatomy and Exercise Basics

*W*hen movement is painful, it's good to know why the heck it's so important to be doing it! Often the first movement is the most painful —and sometimes that's when people want to stop: "Hey, this hurts! Why would I want to do that again?" Short answer: Pain from slow movement is not harmful and it's what we need to do to get better faster.

Moving slowly does not cause injury. As we do a few repetitions we can move easier with less pain. Begin with slow movements in a limited range of motion, then gradually progress toward a full range of motion. Regaining full range of motion might take a few repetitions a day, over a few days, a few weeks, or longer, depending on the severity of the injury. Movement begins slowly, and then we can start moving faster. Once the joint moves well again, soft tissues become healthy and we can have pain relief.

JOINT BASICS

Fibrous joint capsules surround all moveable joints, big and small. The capsules are lined with a soft tissue—synovial membrane (synovium)—that produce synovial fluid (from the word *ovum*, meaning egg) and has a consistency similar to egg whites. Synovial fluid lubricates joint surfaces.

Bursas are soft tissues that surround joints. They are also lined with a synovial membrane and produce synovial fluid to help tendons (fibrous cords connecting muscle to bone) glide and slide over bony prominences around joints.

Synovium in joints and bursas can be injured by poor body mechanics and common strains that cause inflammation. This is known as *synovitis* (swelling of the synovium deep in joints) or *bursitis* (swelling of the synovium superficial to joints). Chronically inflamed synovium is associated with osteoarthritis, the breakdown of cartilage on joint surfaces.

Synovial tissue (both in joints and in bursas) doesn't have a direct blood supply. These soft tissues receive nutrients from fluids passing through them as joints move. They also have a rich network of sensory nerves relaying pain messages to the brain. With immobility, from injury, surgery, extended bed rest, or by avoiding painful movement, joints become less healthy and even more painful to move.

Any joint that's not moving well is going to have sensitive soft tissues around it. This is one good reason why even though a joint is initially painful to move, it needs to move to get these soft tissues and nerves healthy again.

Joint Sounds

Somewhat disturbing can be the sounds that joints make as we move. There are a variety of noises that can come from a joint: Loud clunks, crunchy grinding (*crepitus*), and pops. While moving slowly—and not weight bearing—these sounds are not harmful. A repeated loud joint noise with resistance (lifting weights, doing squats) is not encouraged. Improving mechanics and strengthening around joints (described in the next chapters) will usually quiet them down.

MUSCLE BASICS

Deep muscles are muscles that are close to the bones. These muscles stabilize joints. This has been mentioned a lot regarding the spine. Other joints have deep stabilizing muscles as well. Superficial muscles are layered over deep muscles and are closer to the skin. These muscles move the body.

Muscle strain, or a "pulled" muscle, occurs when a muscle is suddenly overstretched, overworked, or torn. This can happen as a result of fatigue, overuse, overstretching, trauma, or poor body mechanics. After a muscle strain, deep muscles aren't working well and superficial muscles are being overworked, disrupting the coordination of how muscles work together.

A muscle spasm, or cramp, is an abnormal muscle contraction caused by a muscle strain. We are more susceptible to muscle spasms if we are dehydrated. With any muscle strain, there is a lesser or greater degree of muscle spasm involved. A charley horse, or cramp, in the back of the thigh or calf, is a severe spasm affecting the whole muscle or groups of muscles. A milder strain produces a minor spasm in a few muscle fibers.

Breathing deeply and stretching slowly (lengthening the muscle) mechanically allows more blood to flow into the muscle. Followed by using the muscle slowly (contracting or shortening the muscle) and then stretching again, the spasm begins to be relieved. (Slump/PIL is helpful to spinal strains and pains for this reason.)

Spasms are so painful because the muscle in spasm is stuck in a state of contraction and doesn't have blood flowing through it. A muscle needs oxygen to stop contracting. Normal, healthy muscle allows us to move into an end-of-range position and lets us move faster or slower as the situation requires. A muscle in spasm can prevent us from getting to that end-of-range movement when we move slowly—like reaching for that favorite cup on the top shelf with a spasm in the shoulder. It can also prevent us from moving quickly in mid-range—like trying to catch that favorite cup that we didn't quite hold on to.

Chronic muscle strain and spasm can lead to tendonitis—inflammation of the tendon.

NERVE BASICS

Nerve pain signals a problem anywhere along the nerve's path. Pain, tingling, numbness in arms or hands, may originate in the neck, shoulders, elbows, or wrist. Thigh, leg, or foot nerve pain may come from the low back, hip, pelvis, knee, or ankle.

Without oxygen or good blood flow, nerves become irritated and hypersensitive. Beside the unpleasant sensation of pain, we can have other unpleasant sensations from nerves. This can be numbness and tingling, pain, or weird sensations—like the feeling of water trickling over the skin or ants crawling on us.

These sensations are signals to move. We might shake our arms and hands around, or rub the area that feels weird. But there are better ways to give the nerves what they want (Chapter 15).

How Damaged Tissue Heals

In the early stage of healing there is swelling—inflammation—around an injured area. This is the "inflammatory response" to injury. Swelling brings in specialized cells to remove the cells of the damaged or irritated tissue, to begin to replace them with collagen. Collagen is a fibrous connective tissue found throughout the body, whose fibers are highly organized in tendons and ligaments (oriented along lines of stress), and disorganized (crisscrossed) in scar tissue and in early healing. Progressive stretching and strengthening helps to organize collagen fibers after injury. This is key to recovery and good function of healing tissue. It also explains why it's so difficult to begin moving joints that have been immobilized for a length of time—after surgery or a severe injury. The collagen fibers have become more established and thickened in a disorganized pattern from lack of movement.

EXERCISE BASICS

Now we'll go from head to toes with some simple exercises. The idea of all these exercises is to get muscles working well together, joints moving through their full range of motion, and blood flowing to muscles and nerves. This leads to a decrease in pain in order to return to regular activity or exercise—or to begin a more challenging exercise program with a trainer. Again, this is the linking of attention to the moment with action to take when we experience aches and pains. We do this by taking deep breaths to consciously engage a relaxation response as we move—not letting an unconscious, emotional response to pain take over and prevent us from moving. If that happens, we just stop, do some more deep breathing, observe our negative thoughts, and start again with small movement, done even slower.

Be patient. It might take 1-3 days for a minor injury, 2-3 weeks or longer for a moderate or more severe injury. If we can't move easily in a reasonably faster fashion, then we're not quite ready and it will take more time. Just keep at it. If you are not getting better, see a professional. Often, having some manual treatment done (massage therapy, chiropractic, acupressure, physical therapy), can help us to feel better and be able to relax. Exercises for strength and mobility, done after manual treatments, promote longer lasting relief.

Most of these exercises are easy to do during the day, rather than at a special exercise time. Many can be done sitting in the car or at the computer, in bed before going to sleep or before getting up. They can be done as we stand up, sit down or while we're standing or walking.

Do these exercises as you read about them, even if the exercise is for a part of the body where you're not having any problems or have never had a problem: "My feet are fine, I don't need to do this." It won't take long and it's really good to have some idea of how to do these things before you're hurting, so you have the recollection: "Oh, right, I used to be able to do that."

Reminder

- PIL is always the way to start with any problem with the spine (neck, mid-back, low back) as well as any joints that have supporting muscles that connect to the spine (jaw, shoulders, hips).
- If having a problem with one joint, it's a good idea to do all the movements described for that joint and all the movements for the surrounding joints at least once. Continue to do only the movements that are painful or difficult to do.
  - For elbow pain: Do elbow, shoulder, and wrist/hand exercises.
  - For shoulder pain: Do shoulder, neck, and elbow exercises.
  - For knee pain: Do knee, hip, and ankle exercises.
  - For low back pain: Do low back, hip, and mid back exercises.
  - For neck pain: Do neck, shoulder, and mid back exercises.
- The first repetition is usually the worst feeling, and by the last we're moving further with less pain.
- Moving slowly (slowly stretching and contracting muscles) will not cause injury. The unpleasant sensation of pain with slow movement does not equal harm.
- Avoiding movement due to pain is often the start of chronic pain.
- Move slowly through a gradually increasing range of motion. Do 3-5 repetitions holding 3-5 seconds. Do them as needed during the day for temporary pain relief and occasionally to avoid strains.
- Sometimes, fingertip pressure on the area of spasm (the sore spot in the muscle) as we move can allow us to move further. Commercial devices are available—they look like hooked canes or firm small balls for this purpose.
- Once we're doing better with slow movement and isometrics, then we can do movements a little faster.

Chapter 11

All for One and One for All
The Spine: Neck, Mid Back, and Low Back Problems

*P*eople have come to me with stories of their traveling pain. *Not necessarily pain that started when they were traveling— though it might have—but pain that started in their neck. First on the right side, then it moved to the left. A week later the pain had traveled down to the their low back and then up to their mid back. The referral that came from their doctor was for one pain, but really what was bothering them by the time they came in to see me was somewhere else. Neck, mid back, or low back. It's all spinal pain. It all involves postural habits—like doing PIL and Slump/PIL—and body mechanics. But there are some different things to do for self-care that address the unique movement of each area of the spine.*

NECK

With a pain or a "catch" in the neck, a tense muscle has gone into a stronger spasm. We may not be able to turn our head fully. Maybe it's difficult to move in all directions: Looking up, looking down, and turning to look over the shoulder to back up a car. This is something that we want to take care of immediately. It's possible to get back to normal within one to three days.

Neck pain is common with stress related muscle tension. It's not uncommon to think that someone else has caused our neck pain. This stress/pain combo is so common that it even becomes a label for a difficult person: "That guy at work is a pain in the neck." But this is a good time to remember it's only our reaction to someone or some situation that causes the neck to act up. It's the unconscious tensing of muscles when the mind is busy being annoyed. The body is reacting and muscles tense up. When we're not paying attention we have no awareness of what the body is doing. It's good to acknowledge that no one else can actually give us a pain in the neck. At the same time, it's good to be mindful of our thoughts and emotional reactions that have given us a pain in the neck, and address them.

Neck pain can also happen from working in stressful positions—at a computer or working overhead. Another reminder is to do PIL occasionally during the day, especially when working or doing repetitive activities, or doing anything that puts us in an awkward position. If a neck ache or pain is caught early and full range of motion is achieved before going to bed, waking up with a neck in spasm can be avoided altogether.

Stress headaches may be caused by muscle tension in the upper neck—right under the skull. Headaches can be due to other problems: Vascular (too much blood flow in the brain—classic migraine headaches), hormonal, sinus pain, or stress related muscle tension headaches. Treatment of migraines and hormone-related headaches are beyond the scope of this book. However, stress-related or muscle tension headaches come from the muscles of the upper neck and the muscles from the shoulder blades that attach to the neck—the muscles that shrug the shoulders up. The same advice used for neck pain can be applied to muscle tension headaches.

FIRST THING TO DO FOR NECK PAIN

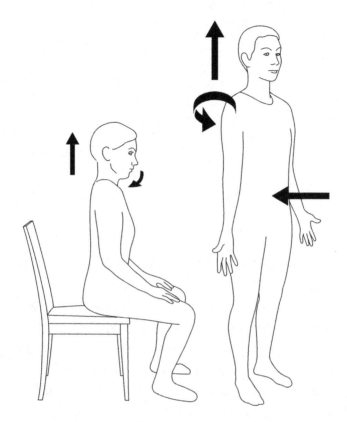

- Lying in bed, standing or sitting: Do PIL, emphasizing the lengthening of the back of the neck (pp. 44, 45, and 49).
- With the back of the neck lengthened, slowly press shoulder blades together and down.
- Hold these positions while taking a few slow, deep breaths (inhale count 2, exhale count 3).

Note: Even with chronic neck pain, doing PIL frequently is the way to begin to get relief.

TILTING HEAD BACK

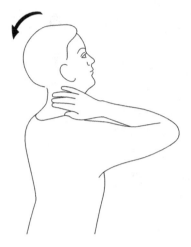

- Sitting or standing in PIL position: Put fingertips on both sides of the neck.
- With light pressure, push under the skull, moving fingertips down the neck, to find the sore spot—where the muscle is in spasm.
- Start again with fingertips right under the skull on the upper neck. Very slowly, tilt the head backward—looking up towards the ceiling—while maintaining gentle pressure with fingertips.
- Stop at the point of increased pain—if there is pain.
- Continue to walk fingertips down the neck about a half inch at a time. Tilt the head backward slowly every time the fingertips move downward.
- When you find a sore spot, repeat 3-5 times slowly, stopping at point of any increased pain.
- Then, return to looking straight ahead in the PIL position. Take a few slow breaths.

TURNING HEAD TO THE SIDE

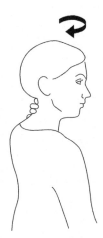

- Sitting or standing in PIL position: Put fingertips of the opposite hand touching the other side of the neck. (For example: Left fingertips on right side of neck.)
- Turn the head slowly—trying to look over the shoulder—while keeping fingertip pressure on the side we're turning towards. (For example: Left fingertips on the right side of neck, head turning to the right.)
- Repeat 3-5 times slowly. Stop at point of any increased pain.
- Return to PIL.
- Do the same, turning the head in the other direction.

TILTING HEAD TO THE SIDE

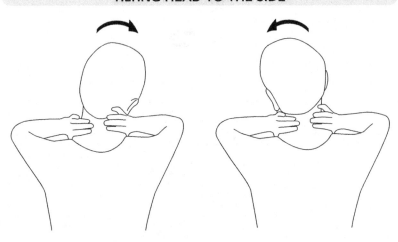

- Sitting or standing in PIL position: Fingertips of both hands touching both sides of the neck.
- Tilt head to the side—ear towards shoulder. Have more fingertip pressure on the side we're tilting towards.
- Repeat 3-5 times slowly. Stop at point of any increased pain.
- Return to PIL.
- Do the same, tilting the head to the other side..

Gradually progress all these movements by slowly doing full range of motion of the neck from the PIL position—turning the head and looking over the shoulder, tilting the head side to side, and tilting the head backward. Do 3-5 times each, every hour—more often if tolerated. Do these movements without using fingertips on the neck as that becomes more comfortable. Keep shoulders down.

LYING ON BACK

- Keep a pillow under the head or go without a pillow if that's more comfortable.

Note: Often a pillow that's too big can give us neck pain. If that's suspect, take away the pillow.

- Lying on back: Do PIL.
- From PIL position roll head side to side.
- If limited in turning neck, place fingertips on both sides of neck and feel for sore spots.
- Then again, slowly roll head side to side with light fingertip pressure on the sore spots.

After getting out of bed continue to do the above movements for neck pain in sitting and standing.

Referred Neck Pain

Referred neck pain is felt in the arms, head, or upper back, coming from a problem in the neck. Disc pain from the neck is often felt between the upper back and the shoulder blade. Or, if nerves from the neck are irritated, it may be felt in the arm. Since these pains often aren't recognized as coming from the neck, all kinds of squirming movements are done to try to relieve them. Twisting and doing prolonged stretches will make things worse. It's good to get into the PIL positions and check neck movement slowly. See if moving the neck makes the upper back or arm pain worse. If it does, then the problem is from the neck.

If neck movement affects these areas of pain, continue to focus on doing PIL throughout the day. Also, it's a good time to review the tips on back support with sitting to more easily keep the pelvis rocked forward and support the affected arm with pillows (pp. 95 and 99). Moving the hand of the affected arm while it's supported, or while walking and doing PIL, helps to get the involved nerves less sensitive.

Anything we do that makes referred pain or numbness worse should be avoided. Especially avoid bringing your chin down to your chest. Continue to return to the PIL position. If doing the PIL position is helpful, even if only at the time we're doing it, we should continue doing PIL as needed. Always be conscious of sitting positions—slump sitting will make these symptoms worse.

Symptoms can be much improved after an hour or so, and much better in one to three days when cared for early. If symptoms haven't improved in this time frame, or if they're getting worse, contact your doctor or health care provider.

CHEST AND MID BACK

Muscle strain and spasm in the thoracic spine—the mid back—can be particularly annoying. So many casual moves affect this area: Sitting and twisting slightly to the side, reaching away from the body, reaching overhead, bending forward, or sideways. Not to mention breathing or sneezing! Sitting can become very uncomfortable with a strain or pain to the mid back. The middle back curves forward slightly, in the opposite direction of the neck and low back. So any slumped sitting can really add to the strain.

If having any chest pain, particularly pain or shortness of breath with activity—like walking, or walking up stairs—call for medical advice. If severe, call for emergency medical assistance (911). It's always good to have the possibility of cardiac or pulmonary symptoms ruled out. But if pain is consistently related to particular movements of the spine, it's safer to say it's from a muscular-skeletal origin. For peace of mind however, always check with a doctor if there's uncertainty.

FIRST THING TO DO FOR MID-BACK PAIN

- Lying down, standing or sitting: Do PIL emphasizing the opening of the chest (pp. 44, 49, 57).
- Accentuate this opening of the chest by slowly pressing shoulder blades together and down.
- Hold these positions while taking a few slow, deep breaths (inhale 2 seconds, exhale 3 seconds).

Diaphragmatic Breathing

The thoracic cage is also known as the rib cage, where the heart and lungs reside. It consists of the 12 thoracic vertebrae (middle back), 12 pairs of ribs, and the sternum (breast bone). That's many moving parts, many little joints.

When we take a deep breath, the primary breathing muscle—the diaphragm (that connects to the lower ribs, lower sternum, and upper lumbar vertebrae)—contracts, rotating ribs outward and downward as lungs expand and fill with air. Secondary muscles can add to the available space for the lungs to expand and elevate the upper ribs. They connect from the upper ribs to the neck, collarbones, and shoulder blades. Under stress, or with pulmonary disease, many of us start using these secondary muscles more than the diaphragm resulting in shallow, upper chest breathing.

We're doing diaphragmatic breathing with comfortable, relaxed breaths, when our shoulders are down—like with PIL—letting the belly and lower ribs expand.

IN SITTING

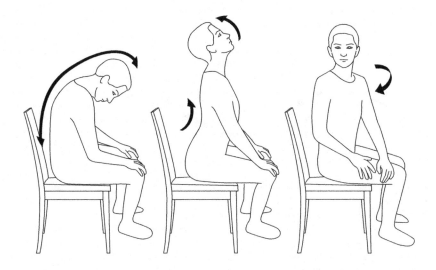

- Round out the middle back slowly. Stop with any increase in pain.
- Slowly straighten back and arch spine backward slowly.
- Repeat 3-5 times and return to PIL.
- From PIL position, slowly turn to one side while maintaining PIL.
- Turn to the other side.
- Repeat 3-5 times and return to PIL.

IN STANDING

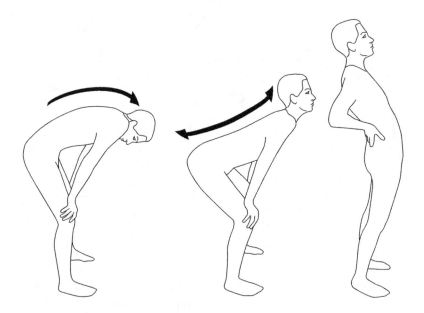

- Have feet spread shoulder width.
- Bend knees and place hands above knees.
- Round up back slowly.
- Let back arch—sag downward—slowly.
- Repeat 3-5 times and return to standing with straight back.
- Stand with hands on waist and slowly arch backward as far as comfortable.
- Return to PIL.

CHEST OPENING

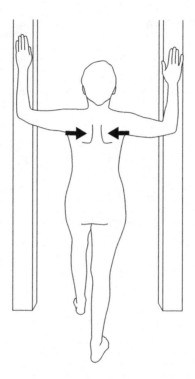

- Stand in open doorway: Hands on doorframe at shoulder height.
- Take a step into doorway, expanding chest and pinching shoulder blades together.
- Repeat 3-5 times.

ON HANDS AND KNEES

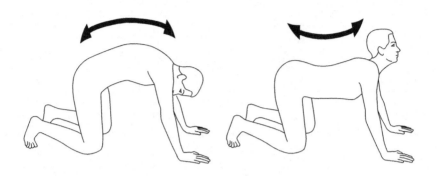

- Let back round up slowly.
- Let back arch—sag downward—slowly.
- Repeat 3-5 times.

Note: This is also known as the cat-camel stretch.

LYING ON SIDE

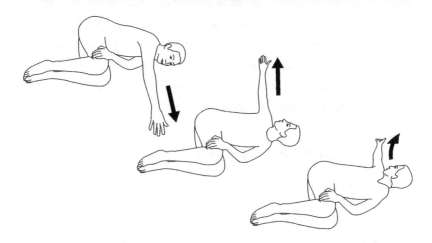

- Bring knees up like in a sitting position.
- Do PIL in side lying, hold 3-5 seconds, and relax.
- Hold upper thigh with lower hand. Slowly reach forward with upper arm.
- Continue to reach forward as arm extends towards ceiling and behind back only as far as comfortable.
- Slowly return in same manner, always reaching long with the arm.
- Repeat 3-5 times.
- Roll onto other side and do the same.

LOW BACK

We know that poor body mechanics can both cause back pain and prevent recovery. For many people just correcting body mechanics and sitting habits—and doing PIL frequently—is the only thing needed to get relief. Too much stretching and twisting in an attempt to get relief, can prolong pain symptoms and should be avoided.

FIRST THING TO DO FOR LOW BACK PAIN

Standing or sitting:
- Do PIL, emphasizing lengthening spine and pulling belly in towards spine.
- Hold while taking a few slow, deep breaths (inhale 2 seconds, exhale 3 seconds).

STANDING

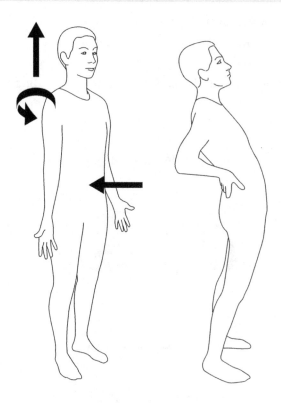

- Standing or sitting: Do PIL (pp.44 and 49).
- Stand with hands on hips and arch backward slightly.
- Walk slowly, with short steps, doing PIL.

SITTING

- Slowly do Slump/PIL (p. 46).
- If too uncomfortable, do PIL in side-lying.
- Continue to do PIL during activity.
- Avoid bending until arching backward in standing is easy and comfortable.

LYING DOWN

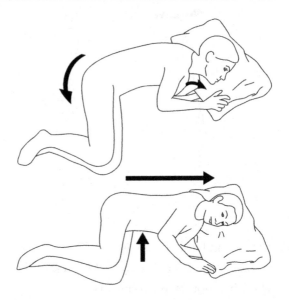

- Lying down on back or side: Do PIL.
- Slowly do Slump/PIL (p. 57). Repeat 3-5 times.

ON HAND AND KNEES

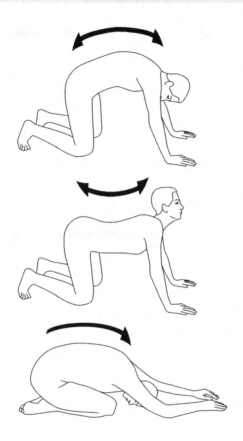

- Let back round up slowly.
- Let back arch—sag downward—slowly.
- Repeat 3-5 times.
- Move into prayer pose, buttocks towards heels, arms reaching forward.

HIP HIKING LYING ON BACK

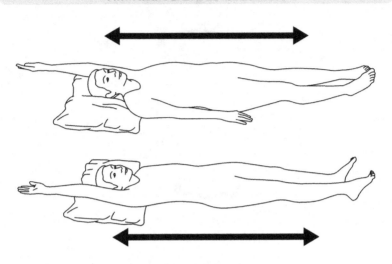

- Lie on back and take a deep breath, then relax.
- Reach long with one leg slowly. Then relax again.
- Reach long with the other leg.
- Move back and forth a few times. (Also good to do with arms overhead, reaching long with the same side arm and leg with the leg rolled inward.)

Note: This is like an exaggerated walking movement without gravity, that gently side bends the low back.

HIP HIKING LYING ON SIDE

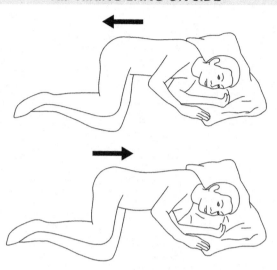

- Lie on side, with knees together or pillow between knees.
- Move pelvis downward towards feet, lengthening the side of the trunk.
- Move pelvis upward towards head, shortening the side of the trunk.
- Repeat 3-5 times.

TRUNK ROTATION

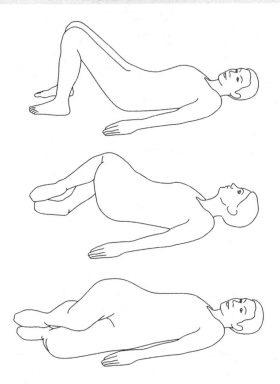

- Lie on back with knees bent and feet flat on bed.
- Rock knees side to side moving slowly.
- Repeat 3-5 times.

Note: For strengthening and stabilizing the low back, see Bridging and Bridging with Marching (pp. 185 and 186).

Reminder

Slump/PIL (Chapter 6) and hip hiking are good to do a few times in bed before going to sleep and before getting up, even when not having pain. It helps maintain good health of spinal joints and good coordination of muscles. It also helps to work out any spinal strain that might have occurred during the day that went undetected, allowing us to wake up pain free—instead of in the grips of spinal muscle spasm!

Chapter 12

Open Wide and Take a Bite
TMJ (Jaw) Problems

A *woman came to see me who had a traumatic injury to her jaw years before that required surgical repair. She had excellent results, leaving her with good contact of her teeth and no complaints of jaw pain afterwards. Gradually, over the few weeks prior to her coming in to the clinic, something had started to change about her jaw that she couldn't understand. Her teeth weren't making good contact anymore. It had become very difficult to chew anything. Her jaw would pop when she tried to open her mouth wide and she was starting to have pain. She was certain that she'd have to have surgery again and had made an appointment with the surgeon she'd seen years before. Her primary care physician suggested she come to see me first.*

I questioned her about what had been going on in her life prior to the change with her bite. She admitted that she'd been under a lot of stress over the past few months. She had changed jobs earlier in the year and was working 12-hour days. Plus, she was a single mom and had to take her child into the ER twice in the past month—once for severe flu symptoms and then a broken arm. She wasn't sleeping well and had started chewing gum a lot—at least 2-3 packs a day. She didn't want to start smoking again!

Fortunately, she didn't need surgery. She just needed to become aware of how stress can affect the jaw. Overworked chewing muscles become strained and go into spasm by unconsciously clenching and grinding teeth—or constantly chewing gum! When TMJ muscles are in spasm on one side, the jaw is pulled to that side. Upper and lower teeth don't line up as usual and the bite is thrown off. As she became more aware of how her body reacted to stress, she began to do relaxation techniques (PIL with deep breathing). She also did the exercises below to get her jaw working right again.

She was an excellent student. Her bite was back to normal in two weeks. Needless to say, she also stopped chewing gum and got more help with stress management.

We talk, sing, yawn, open wide to take a bite, and chew thanks to the temporomandibular (TMJ) joints. That mouthful of a name comes from the meeting of three bones that form two joints. The temporal bones are the part of the skull at the temples. The mandible is the jaw. What's different about the TMJ from other pairs of joints is that a single bone—the mandible—connects two very moveable joints to each other. (Ribs also connect to two joints: The chest bone—the sternum, and the thoracic spine—the middle back. But these joints don't move nearly as much as the TMJs.)

The temporomandibular joints—TMJs—are often the least understood joints of the body. We can feel them move if we put our index fingertips right in front of the little flaps in front of the ear holes (the external auditory meatus). Open your mouth to feel the space made as the mandible, or jaw, rotates downward. We're touching our TMJs.

When we're under excessive stress, the muscles that close the mouth and work to chew food are often strained and go into spasm. Similar to neck pain, this happens when we're unaware of the effect of unconscious stress on the body, as we develop habits of clenching or grinding our teeth during the day. TMJ problems—temporomandibular dysfunction (TMD)—can also be the source of headaches.

Grinding our teeth at night is obviously harder to be conscious of. But if we wake up with a sore jaw, it's easy to suspect that we're either grinding or clenching our teeth as we sleep. We can do pain relieving movements (described below) while we're still in bed. If grinding at night is a habit that can't be broken, many find night guards—soft or firm plastic mouth guards—helpful to protect teeth and prevent the TMJs from being compressed through the night. If an over-the-counter product doesn't help the pain or other symptoms, seek professional advice.

Rest Position of the TMJ

Say the word "mine." The tongue rests on the roof of the mouth on the letter "n". This is the rest position of the TMJs—where the tongue should be all the time when we are not eating, talking, singing, or laughing—when we are standing up, sitting down, or lying down. The tip of the tongue rests on the roof of the mouth with teeth apart. This is also part of the practice of PIL.

It's easy to see how the position of the spine affects the working of the TMJs. Try this: Do PIL with the tongue in the "mine" position and teeth apart, and then slouch down into a slump. As the neck and jaw jut forward, the tongue will leave the roof of the mouth and either "float" in the mouth or touch the back of the lower teeth. This changes the alignment of the TMJs and normal contact of the teeth. If having TMJ pain, it's especially helpful to avoid slouching when chewing.

It's a good practice to start noticing during the day if teeth are touching. This is a great way to begin improving body awareness. If they are touching, it's a good time to do PIL with the TMJ in its rest position.

Popping and Clicking

If TMJs are popping or clicking, muscles surrounding the joints are strained and in some degree of spasm. Sometimes this can happen after a long dentist appointment, excessive gum chewing, or sleeping on the stomach with head turned and jaw shoved off to one side. Often teeth are not making normal contact.

When this is the case, we want to avoid any activities that cause this popping or clicking. Continuing to pop and click won't help anything. Sometimes we have to avoid opening the mouth wide for a while. That includes not eating anything that requires opening wide, like having a big sandwich. Don't eat anything that requires a lot of chewing. Avoid chewing gum. Frequently check for the rest position of the TMJs and return to it as needed.

To improve the movement of opening and closing the mouth without popping or clicking, first look in a mirror. Open the mouth and notice if the jaw shifts to one side or the other. Then work on "Opening the Jaw" (p. 146) followed by "Side-to-Side Movements of the Jaw" (p.147).

FIRST THING TO DO FOR TMJ PAIN

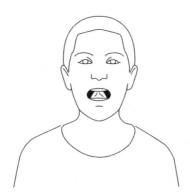

- Do PIL with the tongue on the roof of the mouth, teeth apart.
- Slowly open the mouth, keeping the tongue on the roof of the mouth. Open as wide as possible while still keeping the tongue in place.
- Hold for a few seconds and breathe normally.
- Then let the jaw "float" back upwards, without using any effort to close the mouth.
- Repeat 3-5 times.

Note: This is a simple movement that can prevent TMJ pain from getting worse, or even avoid it altogether.

To be less conspicuous— so people don't think you've gotten really weird and fish-like opening your mouth for no good reason— this can be done with just slightly opening the mouth, without separating the lips.

Some people's lips don't close easily because of the way they're built. This can still be done without separating the lips any further.

Some people's tongues aren't able to rest in this position—some tongues are shorter than others. But still, teeth shouldn't touch unless we're chewing.

OPENING THE JAW

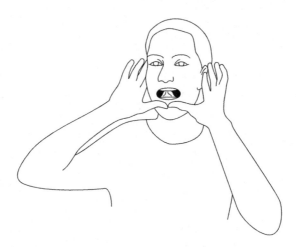

- In front of a mirror, do PIL with the tongue on the roof of the mouth.
- Place index fingers on both TMJs, in front of ear flaps.
- Place tips of thumbs together, on the chin, just below the lower lip.
- Open the mouth, keeping the tongue on the roof of the mouth as long as possible. Gently use a very light pressure of the thumbs to guide the chin downward as the mouth opens wider. (Often the problem is that the jaw is jutting forward as the mouth starts to open. Thumbs on the chin prevent that forward shift.)
- If the jaw shifts to one side, or the TMJs pop or click, stop at that point and relax, letting the jaw float back up to a rest position.
- Stop short of any shift or pop or click.
- If you can do this easily, with the help of the thumbs, guide the chin straight down as you open wider allowing the tongue to leave the roof of the mouth, without clicking or popping.
- Then guide the chin back upwards, tongue back in the rest position. (There's no need to hold the open mouth position.)
- Repeat 3-5 times.

SIDE TO SIDE MOVEMENTS OF THE JAW

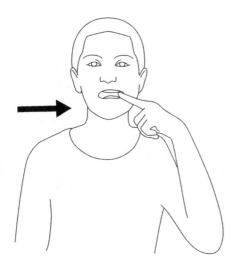

- Still looking in mirror, do PIL. Put the tip of the index finger on the upper teeth, in front of the molars—the teeth in the back of the mouth. Don't try to keep the tongue on the roof of the mouth.
- Shift the jaw sideways so lower teeth touch the fingertip. Try doing this on the other side. If there's no discomfort and the jaw moves easily side to side, then that movement is not a problem.
- If this is a problem, do these sideways movement 3-5 times slowly, to start. Stop short of any clicking or popping.
- Continue doing this until teeth are making good contact again.

Reminder

If TMD (temporomandibular dysfunction) symptoms have gone on for a while—3-6 months—it might take between two to six weeks to improve completely. For more severe TMJ pain, gently brushing an ice cube over the joint for up to one minute, 1-3 times a day after doing exercises can be helpful.

Being aware of the rest position of the jaw—teeth apart and tongue on the roof of the mouth—can prevent any TMD from ever developing. If problems are caught early, TMD can improve in just a few days.

Chapter 13

Reaching for the Stars
Shoulder, Elbow, Wrist, and Hand Problems

*T*here are many ways that arms and hands can be strained
and become painful. But it often boils down to one of a few
possible scenarios:

- *Doing something for too long—overuse and muscle strain—or using poor body mechanics.*
- *Doing a quick movement with the arm extended from the body—especially one that we haven't warmed up for or practiced.*
- *Having the arm in an awkward position for too long when sitting or sleeping.*
- *Experiencing some kind of trauma—a strain from a fall, breaking a bone, recovering from surgery*

We can plow along with minor shoulder, elbow, or hand pain. We might start doing things differently—how we put on a jacket;

or avoid other things—stop doing fine work with our hands. We get along pretty well until one day we turn a key just the wrong way, or use a pair of scissors, and we wince—or holler! Reaching forward or overhead is miserable, if not impossible. Sleeping becomes a nightmare. Things can quickly get out of hand. But they don't have to.

The Amazing and Vulnerable Shoulder Joint

How can a joint be so mobile without falling apart and getting injured? The collarbone connecting to the sternum in the chest and the acromion process—a boney prominence of the shoulder blade—adds stability to the joint while still allowing the shoulder to have a lot movement. The shoulder is a ball and socket joint. The socket is made deeper by the labrum, a rubbery fibro-cartilage around the edge of the joint surface on the shoulder blade—the glenoid fossa. The ball is the head of the humerus—the long bone of the upper arm.

Like all moveable joints, shoulders are held together with ligaments—bone-to-bone fibrous tissue— and a joint capsule. What really keeps the shoulder stabile and functioning well is its musculature. The rotator cuff muscles, the deep stabilizers of the shoulder joint, work in coordination with the superficial muscles surrounding the joint. They make safe movement of the shoulder possible.

The tendons of the rotator cuff muscles attach deeply around the joint capsule of the shoulder. The muscles themselves attach directly on the shoulder blade. Pinching the shoulder blades together and down—like in PIL—is an isometric contraction of these muscles and initiates good contact between the joint surfaces of the shoulder. When these deep muscles are weakened by strain or deconditioning, a joint that depends greatly on muscles for stability can easily be injured. To strengthen them, we can pinch the shoulder blades back and down occasionally as we work—while our arms are forward, at our sides, or overhead.

This is why doing PIL is the first step to addressing any problem with the shoulder. In addition to lengthening the spine and isometric strengthening for deep abdominal and neck muscles, PIL also—by pinching shoulder blades together and down—is an isometric for the deep muscles of the shoulder.

SHOULDERS

Shoulders are the most moveable joints in the human body. They're mobile enough to reach way overhead or allow us to scratch between the shoulder blades. We lift things overhead—heavy weights, if we're strong enough. We can swing arms around like a goofy kid or do impressive gymnastic moves. The human shoulder, along with those of other primates, is an evolutionary marvel.

Shoulders are often strained by having them too rounded forward as we work, drive, and sit at the computer. Sometimes that might be a habitual posture that's never bothered us. It doesn't bother us until we've strained the shoulder with an awkward reach behind the body, or as we try to quickly catch something falling away from the body. Other times, shoulders are injured by habits like sitting with an elbow out the window when we're driving, or sleeping using the arm as a pillow with the shoulder pinched up to the ear.

With poor coordination of the deep muscles of the shoulder, we start to use the arm awkwardly in an attempt to avoid pain. I've heard horrific noises come from chronically strained shoulders and have personally felt the sharp, knife-like pain that comes from moving in the wrong direction with an acutely strained shoulder. Guess what? We do the same thing for either problem.

Shoulder Impingement

The subacromial space of the shoulder is formed between the upper shoulder blade (the acromion) and the upper arm (the head of the humerus). Rotator cuff tendons and the subacromial bursa are between these bones. With tendonitis or a subacromial bursitis, painful soft tissue is "pinched" between the bones with reaching forward or outward. This is known as shoulder impingement. Pinching shoulder blades together and down with palms forward (PIL) makes this space bigger. If caught early, doing shoulder stretches, elastic band exercises (pp. 158-160), and frequently doing PIL, can improve this condition quickly.

FIRST THING TO DO FOR SHOULDER PAIN

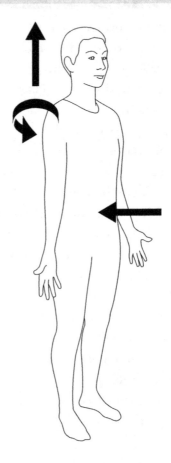

- Sitting or standing: Bring arms to sides with palms forward and do PIL (pp. 44, 45, and 49).
- Emphasize pinching the shoulder blades together and down.
- If carrying weight or working with arms forward, overhead, or while pushing or pulling, simply pinch shoulder blades together and down as you lengthen the spine—as well as you can—as you continue working.

SHOULDER STRETCHES

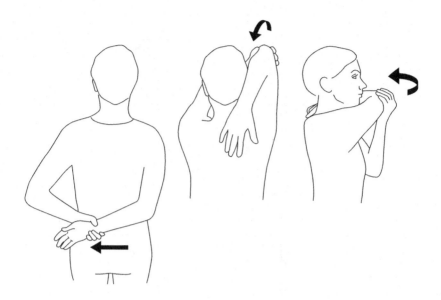

- Reach hand behind back. Grab the wrist with the other hand and pull across the back. If it's difficult to grab the wrist, use a towel behind the back to pull the arm.
- Reach hand behind the head and push elbow up trying to get arm to the side of the head and fingertips down the spine.
- Reach across to the other shoulder, pushing elbow with the other hand. Try to push the arm towards front of the neck.
- After stretching, pinch shoulder blades together back and down doing PIL.
- Do stretches in sequence 1-3 times holding a few seconds each.

Note: For shoulder pain after stretching, use ice (p. 103) in sitting (p. 99).

ACTIVE ASSISTED RANGE OF MOTION: FINGER WALK UP WALL

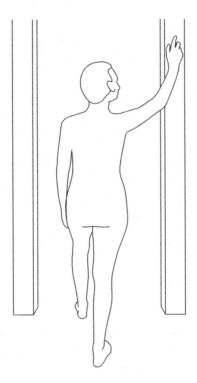

Active assisted exercises are used for shoulder stiffness, weakness, or after surgical procedures.

- Stand in a doorway with fingertips on door-frame or wall.
- Walk fingers up the wall, stepping in closer to the wall, as the arm gets higher.
- Slowly walk fingers back down, stepping back.
- Repeat 5-10 times.

ACTIVE ASSISTED RANGE OF MOTION: CANE EXERCISE

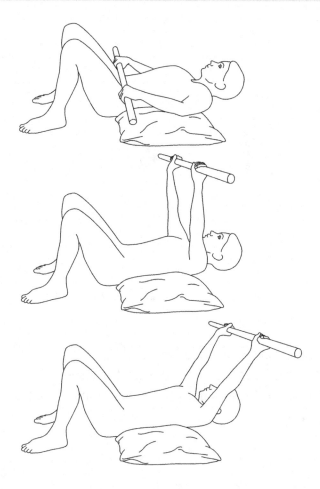

- Lie on back holding cane—or broomstick handle—with both hands.
- Raise arms up towards ceiling, reaching upwards, bringing shoulder blades forward.
- Slowly bring arms overhead.
- Return arms towards ceiling and then down to side. Easier on the shoulder to bend elbows, bringing them back to side.
- Repeat 5-10 times.

SHOULDER ROLLS

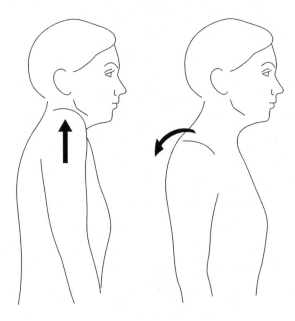

- Shrug shoulders up toward ears.
- Bring shoulders back and down in a half circle.
- End by pinching shoulder blades together back and down, do-
  ing PIL.
- Relax.

SHOULDER BLADE EXERCISE

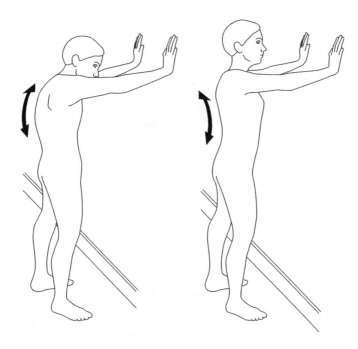

- Facing a wall, extend arms shoulder height and put palms on wall.
- Push away from wall, rounding out upper back— shoulder blades moving forward.
- Keeping arms straight, move chest forward.
- Pinch shoulder blades together.
- Move back and forth 3-5 times.

ELASTIC BAND STRENGTHENING: BASIC PULL

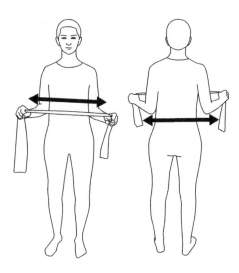

Note: The only exercise equipment recommended in this book is elastic exercise bands. These are just great for shoulder, elbow, and wrist strengthening. They can be purchased online or in sport stores and come in a variety of strengths. Resistance of the bands varies with color.

- Stand in PIL position: Hold elastic exercise band with both hands, elbows at waist.
- Pinch shoulder blades back and down. Keep elbows in towards waist.
- Slowly pull hands apart, short of any pain. Hold position with band stretched for 3-5 seconds.
- Slowly return. Repeat 3-5 times.

ELASTIC BAND STRENGTHENING: OVERHEAD PULL

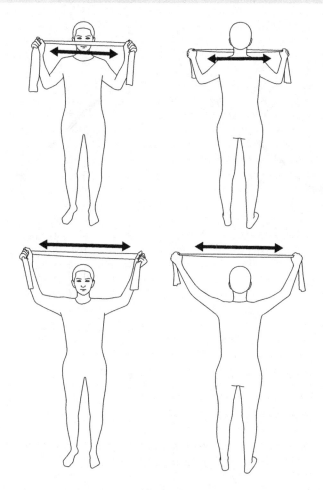

- Stand in PIL position and do Basic Pull.
- Emphasize pinching shoulder blades together.
- Raise hands overhead while continuing to pull band with hands outward.
- Only go as far as comfortable.
- Keep pulling band outward with hands as arms are lowered.
- When elbows have returned to waist, relax.
- Repeat 3-5 times slowly.

ELASTIC BAND STRENGTHENING: DIAGONAL PULL

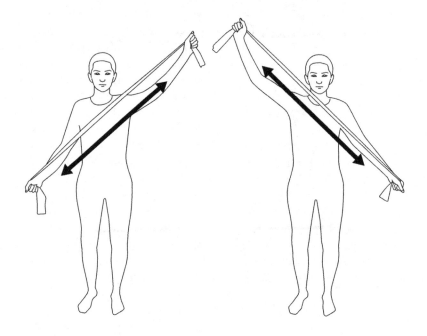

- Stand in PIL position and do Basic Pull.
- Pull elastic exercise band diagonally.
- Repeat 3-5 times slowly.

Note: Use elastic exercise bands as needed throughout day for pain relief and for improving strength and coordination.

Note: To avoid shoulder strain when pulling the cord of a chainsaw, mower, or weed whacker, remember to pinch the shoulder blade back as you pull the cord.

Frozen Shoulder

Many of us have heard of a "frozen" shoulder, also known as adhesive capsulitis. It is a fairly common—but not a well understood— condition, involving a thickening of the joint capsule. It occurs in women more often than men, usually from middle age and onward. It can sometimes occur after shoulder surgeries. It's more frequently seen in post-menopausal women and may have a hormonal connection. The frozen shoulder comes on suddenly, limiting movement. It starts off extremely painful, and then becomes less painful but stays stuck. We can't move the shoulder and someone else can't move it for us.

Here's another personal story. I developed the beginnings of a frozen shoulder. Quite suddenly I realized that I didn't have full range of motion reaching behind my back or overhead. Any fast movement with that arm away from my body was very painful. It was knee-buckling painful. I began strengthening exercises with the elastic bands (pp. 158-160) along with gentle stretching (p.153), a few repetitions as needed for pain during the day, and doing PIL frequently. This quickly thawed the early stages of a frozen shoulder. (Good to point out that the elastic band exercises relieved the pain immediately, but temporarily, during those few days of having a frozen shoulder. I used the band for a few repetitions, almost every hour.)

My shoulder was better within a few days. Very different from more typical frozen shoulder stories that can take up to six months to two years to completely recover, if it does completely recover. This is a very dramatic case of how catching something early, and not avoiding a little pain, can make all the difference in the world.

Note: Odd thing about the more typical long lasting frozen shoulder: Final recovery can sometimes be just as sudden as the onset of the problem. After six months or even two years of doing painful stretching and living with a stiff shoulder, one day it suddenly is better.

ELBOWS, WRISTS, AND HANDS

Sometimes a client with a hangdog look on their face would come in to the clinic wearing funky, dirty, old wrist braces or elbow straps. This was quite challenging. First I had to convince them that wearing all those things was not helping them. "What do you mean?" they'd say defensively. "I can't work without them. I work on a computer for eight hours a day."

Braces and straps are often what a doctor or physical therapist recommends initially for strains to the elbow, wrist, or hand. These should only be used for work or sleep, if needed, and taken off at least a few times during the day for range of motion and strengthening. Some people just leave them on. It's very painful to begin to do range of motion exercises after being immobilized. When they finally try to take them off, the pain has gotten much worse. So back on they go. By and by, the braces and straps are older, funkier, and dirtier, and elbows, wrists, and hands are stiffer and weaker.

Usually as we work, elbows are bent, wrists ideally are straight, and fingers and thumbs are gripping or pushing something. Repetitive work and prolonged work positions cause muscles to be overworked in one direction and to become weakened in the other. To relieve the strain of repetitive work we need to do the opposite movements throughout our workday.

We can do these movements the moment we feel the least amount of strain, ache, or pain. We can take little breaks as we work, play, and create. Breaks don't mean we have to stand up and walk around—though both are good things to do if we've been sitting for much longer than an hour. We can just do PIL, pinch the shoulder blades together, and then move elbows, wrists, and hands around. Get the blood flowing. Get the muscles working.

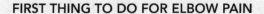

FIRST THING TO DO FOR ELBOW PAIN

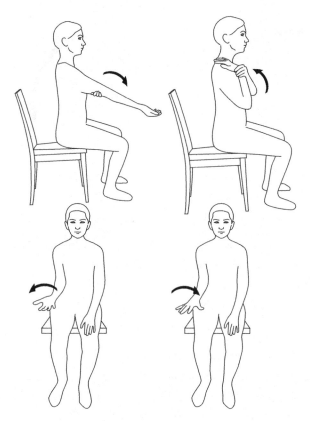

Begin by doing PIL in standing or sitting, slowly straightening the elbow.

- Straighten the elbow slowly, relax and straighten again until able to fully straighten it.
- Bend elbow. Turn palm upward and then downward. Relax and repeat until able to fully turn palm up and down.
- Bend elbow with palm turned upward and then straighten.
- Bend elbow with palm turned downward and then straighten.
- Repeat until full range of motion is restored.

Note: Often a bent elbow is painful when sleeping. To avoid this, wear an elastic sleeve over the elbow. The firm pressure keeps the elbow from being comfortable fully bent. A tight sock with the foot cut out can work as well.

FIRST THING TO DO FOR WRIST/HAND/THUMB PAIN

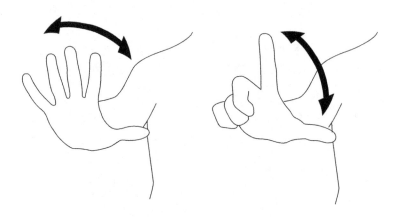

- Open hand, fingers spread wide and wrist pulled back as if signaling to a distant waiter for a "table for five." Relax. Repeat until full range of motion is restored.
- Especially focus on the thumb, trying to make an "L" between the index finger and thumb with wrist pulled back.

Note: Making an "L" between the thumb and index finger stretches the muscles at the base of the thumb. Without doing this stretch these muscles shorten and over time the thumb will gradually rotate inward towards the palm. This can cause osteoarthritis, a common and painful problem with thumbs. It's important to frequently stretch the thumb out fully several times, holding a few seconds or longer as needed for pain and after working and gripping with the hands. See more movements for arms in Nerve Problems (Chapter 15).

STRETCHES FOR WRIST AND FINGER JOINTS

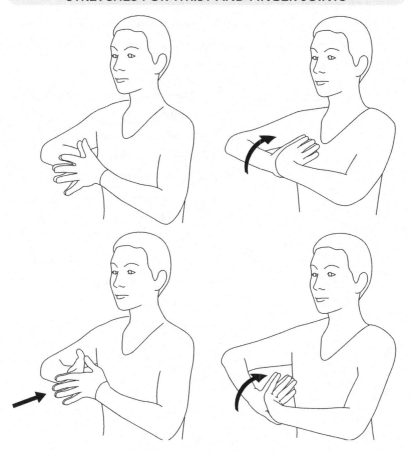

- Place palms together with arms extended straight out from the chest.
- Keep the palms together and bend elbows.
- Bring hands close to the chest.
- Hold a few seconds and then go back and forth.
- When this is comfortable, bring hands close to the chest and rotate the forearms so fingertips point toward the chest.
- Rotate so fingertips are pointing away from the chest.
- To stretch fingers, do the same thing, but this time, let the palms separate and keep fingers together as hands come in toward the chest. Rotate forearms with fingertips pointing toward the chest, then away from the chest.

STRETCHES FOR FOREARM/HAND MUSCLES & TENDONS

The muscles and tendons of the forearm and hand cross over a lot of joints. To stretch the forearm muscles well, we also need to include the hands in the stretch.

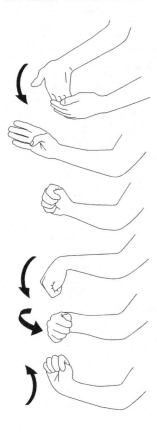

- With the elbow bent at the side, have the palm turned upward.
- Pull down on the finger tips, stretching the palm and forearm.
- Make a fist with thumb in the palm and fingers wrapped around the thumb.
- Move the fist downward in toward the forearm.
- Continue to move the fist in a circle.
- Do this with the elbow bent and with the elbow straight.
- Repeat 3-5 times.
- Follow by opening the hand and spread fingers out straight and wide, doing "table for five."

GRIP STRENGTH

- To work on grip strength, push the tip of the thumb into the tips of the other fingers of the same hand. Going back and forth across all the fingers can start to get our grip strength back.
- Strengthen hands by gripping fingertips and tip of the thumb into a firm or slightly pliable ball that fits into the hand. Grip and hold a few seconds, relax and follow with the "table for five" stretch.
- Repeat 3-5 times.

Hand Work

Usually, as we use our hands, we're gripping, holding, or pushing something with the fingertips. (When gripping or pushing with the thumb, use the tip of thumb, not the pad, to avoid joint stress.) Unless we purposefully do it, we usually aren't stretching the fingers and thumb out straight. Pulling hands back and straightening the fingers and thumb—"table for five" and making an "L" between index finger and thumb (p. 164)—is good to do during, and after doing, any prolonged work with the hands, even if we're not feeling pain.

Moving into these stretch positions, we're stretching strained muscles by using the opposite—often weaker—muscles. If a strain is caught early enough, sometimes that's all it takes to improve. Hold the hand in the "table for five" position for a few seconds. Relax and repeat a few times.

ELASTIC BAND STRENGTHENING: WRIST

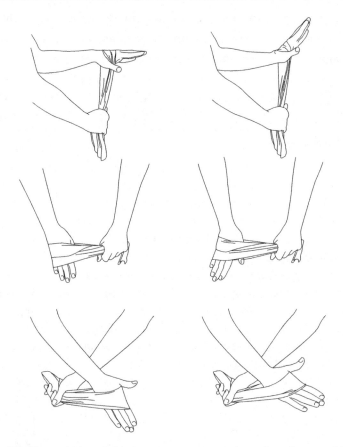

- Hold single band for less resistance, or loop band around hand for more resistance.
- Keep wrist straight against resistance. Begin with isometric contractions—strengthening without movement (pictures on left).
- Pull elastic using other hand for 4 directional strengthening:
    1. Back of hand upwards, pull down.
    2. Palm upwards, pull down (p. 169).
    3. Pull away from little finger.
    4. Pull away from thumb.
- Hold 5-10 seconds. Repeat 3-5 times.
- Then move wrist against resistance (pictures on right).

ELASTIC BAND STRENGTHENING: BENDING ELBOW

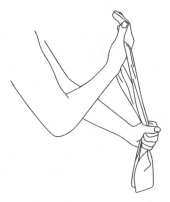

• Hold elastic exercise band in both hands with elbows straight.
• Slowly bend one elbow, keeping wrist straight.
• Hold 5-10 seconds. Relax.
• Repeat 3-5 times.

ELASTIC BAND STRENGTHENING: STRAIGHTENING ELBOW

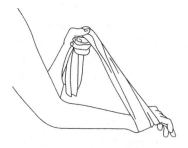

• Hold the band in both hands with elbows bent.
• Slowly straighten one elbow, keeping wrist straight.
• Hold 5-10 seconds. Relax.
• Repeat 3-5 times.

Tennis and Golfer's Elbow

Tennis and golfer's elbow occur most frequently in people who have never played tennis or golf. But the names have stuck. Often we strain forearms and hands by doing repetitive work. They could more accurately be called carpenter's, plumber's, or gardener's elbows.

Though the pain is around the elbow, it's the muscles of the forearm that have been strained. Remember that muscles develop varying degrees of spasm from overuse. Do all the movements listed under "First Thing to Do for Painful Elbows" and "First Thing to Do for Wrists/Hands/Thumbs," but especially the ones when making a fist. Rotate the wrist and then do the "table for five" stretch.

Odds are we'll find a particular movement more difficult and painful. This is the one we need to work on. If we intervene early and take the time to do these exercises whenever we feel pain in the elbow and forearm, we can avoid chronic conditions. If we already have a chronic pain condition, these stretches will improve it. If we need to, we can find the sore spots in the forearm that are in spasm. Put fingertip pressure on the spot and then do the same moves again. Do these exercises a few times during and after work, while we're relaxing in the evening, and before bed and in the morning.

To repeat the most important point: The most difficult movement to do is the one to keep working on. Keep moving slowly, doing a few repetitions, until that movement feels better.

Protect Hands/Use Tools

Fingers have small joints, and small joints are vulnerable to side-to-side stress and strain. Osteoarthritis—wear and tear of joint surfaces—is common in the hand due to sideways strains to the joints. It's best to keep joints straight and not bent sideways. Trying to open a stuck jar, for instance, twists finger joints to the side. It's a good idea to have some handy tools around the kitchen (or wherever needed) that can be used in the palm with a more open grip to prevent twisting strains to the fingers.

Trigger Finger

Something can happen to fingers which is quite uncomfortable. Fingers can get "stuck." Usually they're bent and if we try to straighten them it's incredibly painful, and scary, too. Scary because we expect that pulling them straight would make them feel better. But it doesn't. The fingers are really difficult and painful to straighten.

This is called "trigger finger." It happens when the long tendons of the fingers get stuck in the tendon sheaths they move through. The forearm muscles are often in spasm. To prevent this, keep hands healthy by doing all the stretches mentioned.

But if this does happen, there's an easy way to fix it. Let's

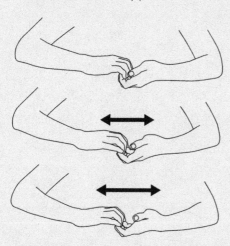

say a finger is stuck in a bent position and won't straighten out. Instead of trying to pull the fingers out straight, do "fingertip wrestling." Hook fingertips into the fingertips of the other hand. Grip with the fingertips as strongly as we can. Continue to hold this grip and slowly let the fingers become straighter. This is sort of like losing an arm wrestling match. As the fingers straighten, just as suddenly that horrible pain is gone. Good to do a big "table for five" stretch afterward, and then slowly move the hand in a partial fist and do the fingertip wrestling again. Go back and forth a few times until able to make a full fist and open the hand wide without a problem.

This can also be done gripping into a ball and slowly releasing, if gripping fingertips is too difficult. Then doing the "table for five" stretch (p. 164).

After experiencing "trigger finger" even once, you'll be only too happy to do the hand and wrist stretches.

> **Reminder**
>
> Work, play, and creative endeavors can distract us from paying attention to the body's aches and pain. It's good to remember that we live through the body, not in spite of it. Awareness and kindness goes a long way with how we treat ourselves.
>
> Refer to Chapter 15 "The Nerve of it All" about neural mobilization to put the finishing touch on any arm exercises.

Chapter 14

From the Ground Up
Hip, Knee, Ankle, and Foot Problems

I saw a woman one day who was scheduled to have a knee re-placement surgery the next week. She had the typical-looking knee that's about to undergo this kind of procedure. She couldn't straighten it completely and it looked puffy. She walked with a cane. I was seeing her for neck pain, but I asked what kind of injury she'd originally had to her knee.

I was surprised to hear that the only injury she'd ever had was some kind of knee bursitis years before. Painful swelling around her kneecap had kept her from trying to straighten it out. She never went to get any help from professionals. She just kept walking around on a slightly bent knee because it felt better to walk like that at the time.

Walking like this changes the dynamics of weight bearing throughout the body. When knees—or hips—don't straighten completely, we start bearing weight on joint surfaces that aren't optimal for full weight bearing. Cartilage on joint surfaces eventually

173

wears and breaks down over time. Then we have arthritis. After six months or more the soft tissues surrounding a joint get shortened and thickened, developing a contracture—a permanent lack of flexibility in a joint that becomes essentially stuck in a limited range.

It's the same old story. First, she didn't realize how important it was to get her knee to straighten completely. She didn't want to do something that was painful. She didn't understand that the pain would improve by doing some initially uncomfortable exercise. She was unaware that changing how she walked would have unforeseen consequences. This contracture gave her a "functionally" shorter leg. If we bend a knee slightly, the length of that leg shortens. If just one knee is bent and we walk around like that for years, the spine starts to develop a sideways curve as a compensation for the shorter leg.

I was seeing her for neck pain that started to bother her after years of back pain. The back pain started after her knee pain. The knee pain started with something simple and easily fixable that was unknown to her. This is a cautionary tale. Don't let it happen to you! If you've gotten this far in the book, it won't.

Measurable Leg Length Difference

If we do have an actual leg length difference—bones are different lengths—it's good to have a professional assess it and add a lift in one shoe to compensate for it. Rule of thumb: Never over-correct the shorter leg. It's usually best to under-correct it slightly to avoid back problems.

HIPS

If the TMJ is the least understood joint, then hip joints are a close second. Many people don't even know where the hip joint is. The confusion about where the joint is located is most likely due to the misnomer that when we ask someone to "put your hands on your hips" or in sports to "swing through with your hips"— we're actually talking about the pelvis. So many times someone would come in the clinic with "hip pain," and when asked to show exactly where the pain was, they'd reach around and touch their sacrum or buttock. Nope. That area is considered "back pain." When the hip joint is the culprit, we usually feel the pain in the groin or down the front of the thigh.

Another common spot to have hip pain is at the upper, outer side of the thigh. The greater trochanter is the bony prominence on the femur (the outer and upper thigh) with lots of muscular attachments and a big bursa. Hip bursitis usually involves the trochanter and can become very painful, especially with side-lying, sitting, and walking.

The hip is a very mobile joint—think ballerinas and gymnasts—but unlike the shoulder joint, it also bears a lot of weight. Problems like osteoarthritis occur when we lose flexibility and strength around a joint. In the hip the most common muscles to lose their flexibility are the hip flexors. These are the muscles that lift the leg when we're going up stairs or up a hill, or when we're swinging the leg forward while taking a step. They're the muscles that are in a shortened position when we sit. If we sit a lot and take fairly short steps when we walk, it's easy for this muscle to stay shortened.

The hip flexor muscles attach deep to the internal organs on the upper lumbar vertebrae and to the inner part of the upper thigh (the lesser trochanter). To do an effective stretch the pelvis needs to rock backward with the hip turned inward. This pelvic position is the opposite of PIL. Another good reason why hip flexors get shortened—stretching them is kind of awkward!

FIRST THING TO DO FOR HIP PAIN

- Stand and do PIL (p. 49).
- Emphasize tightening the buttocks and pulling the belly in towards the spine.
- Walk slowly with attention to foot contact on the ground, knee bending over foot (pp. 84 and 85).

Hip Joint Anatomy

Hip joints are pretty much in the middle of the groin. Right where we bend when sitting. It's where the thigh bone—the femur—meets up with the pelvis—the acetabulum. The acetabulum is the socket for this ball and socket joint. It's where the three bones of the pelvis—the pubic, ilium, and ischium—come together. Like the shoulder joint, the socket is made deeper by a labrum, a rubbery fibro-cartilage on the edge of its circumference. For mobility, the hip also comes in second after the shoulder.

HIP FLEXOR STRETCH

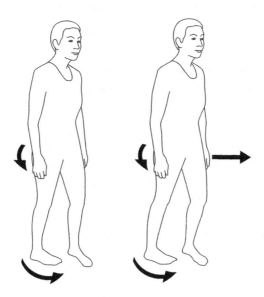

- Hold onto something for balance if needed.
- Feet shoulder width apart, bring one foot back so that tip of the big toe is even with the heel of the other foot.
- Turn the back foot inward—toe inward, heel outward (pigeon toed).
- Shift weight to the back foot.
- Tuck pelvis to flatten back, opposite of PIL. (If you need help with getting this, practice by standing with back against a wall, bend knees slightly and press low back into the wall, doing a pelvic "tuck.")
- Keep pelvis in this position. Slowly shift weight onto the front leg.
- A pull should be felt in the groin area of the leg in back.

Note: The weight shift forward for the final part of the stretch is a small movement.

Other tricky stretches for the hips are for the outside of the hip and thigh. These are good for pain around the greater trochanter, the bony prominence on the outer part of the upper thigh. This area can be under stress from poor body mechanics—less often trauma—and can develop trochanteric bursitis.

On the side of the hip is the ilio-tibial band (ITB)—a broad flat tendon attached to the tensor fascia lata (TFL). This muscle lies between the trochanter and the iliac crest where we "put our hands on our hips." The broad flat tendon of the ITB is along the outer thigh, extending to the outer part of the knee. If you're not having pain in this area, this description is probably at least giving you a headache.

Osteoarthritis of the Hip and Knee

Osteoarthritis is common in hip and knee joints. Both are large weight bearing joints and develop osteoarthritis from the wear-and-tear breakdown of the cartilage covering the joint surfaces. A combination of problems can lead to osteoarthritis:

1. Poor flexibility of the joints themselves due to thickening and poor health of the synovium (p. 112).
2. Limited flexibility of the muscles around the joints.
3. Poor body mechanics—awkward angles as we bear weight.
4. Weakness and poor joint stability.
5. A history of trauma.

The best treatment for osteoarthritis in any joint is to regain and maintain as much flexibility and strength around the joint as possible. It's important to keep moving but with lower impact activities—walking and biking instead of running and jumping. Osteoarthritic joints need to have their range of motion maintained, or regained, to maximize flexibility of surrounding muscles.

Not moving arthritic joints—by letting pain run the show—is one of the worst things to do. That leads to more pain. This in part explains the high number of hip and knee joint replacements we see today. The 1 million annual operations are expected to increase substantially to 4 million by 2030.*

* Kurtz S, Song K, Lau E, Mowat F, Halpern M. *Projecting of primary and revision hip and knee arthroplasty in the United States 2005-2030*. Journal of Bone and Joint Surgery Am. 2007;89(4):780.

ITB (ILIO-TIBIAL BAND) STRETCH: EASIER

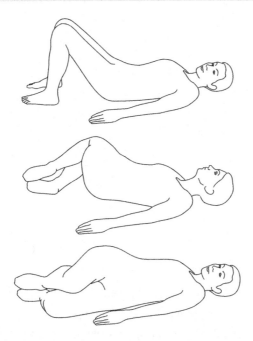

- Knees bent and feet flat on the bed or floor.
- Have feet shoulder width apart.
- Bring knees down to one side while keeping the upper back and shoulders still. Feel the stretch on the outer thigh of the upper leg and the same side of the trunk.
- Hold a few seconds and breath.
- Then bring the knees back to the starting position and go to the other side. This also gives a gentle twist to our spines. (Only go as far with the knees as is comfortable if we're having back pain. It's always better to begin with small movements.)
- Repeat 3-5 times.
- Relax.

ITB (ILIO-TIBIAL BAND) STRETCH: STRONGER

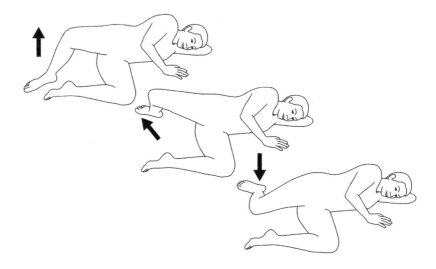

- Lie on the less painful side to start. Have knees pulled up like in a sitting position. Use a pillow between the knees (not in illustration).
- With the painful leg upward, keep feet together and lift up the knee.
- Slide that foot backwards on the bed or floor until the upper hip is straight—like in standing. The knee stays up and bent as the foot slides backwards.
- Stay lying on side. Don't roll backwards as the leg is moving back.
- When the hip is straight, lower the knee. This stretches the outer hip.
- Go slowly and hold for a few seconds. Breathe.
- To get out of this position, lift the knee up again, keeping the foot down, and slide that leg back to the pillow between the knees, feet together.
- Repeat 3-5 times.
- If painful after stretching, lie on the non-painful side with a pillow between the knees and apply an ice pack for 10 to 15 minutes.
- Do the stretch on the other side if lying on the painful side is tolerated. This will show how a hip that's not sore should feel.

INNER THIGH STRETCH

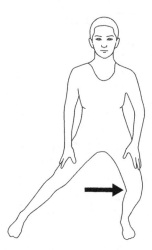

- Take a wide step sideways.
- Keep pelvis level with the ground and lunge sideways, stretching the inner thigh of the leg with the knee straight.
- Feet can be facing forward to begin, and then rotate the hip of the extended leg by turning the foot inward and outward, to stretch different parts of the muscles.

The Piriformis Muscle

The piriformis is a deep stabilizing muscle of the hip joint. It attaches from the front of the sacrum—lowest part of the spine— and the greater trochanter—outer and upper part of the thigh. For extra trouble, the sciatic nerve (of sciatica fame) crosses below this muscle in the buttock. Yes, it's the proverbial pain in the ass. Strain and spasm in the piriformis can set off what's known as a "piriformis syndrome," which can feel just like sciatica from the low back. This pain can be felt in the back and side of the thigh, leg, and/or foot. Maintaining flexibility of the hip and using good body mechanics can prevent pain problems and strengthen muscles.

BUTTOCK STRETCH: EASIER

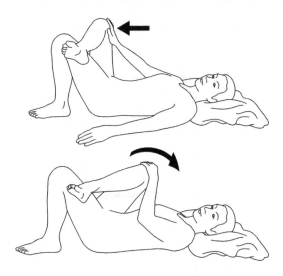

- Knees bent and feet flat on the bed or floor.
- Cross one ankle on other knee.
- Push crossed knee downward toward feet.
- Pull crossed knee upward toward opposite shoulder.
- Hold 3-5 seconds. Relax.
- Repeat 3-5 times.

Body Mechanics and Hip Pain

Review the chapter on Body Mechanics (Chapter 7). Poor body mechanics causes hip pain and prevents recovery. Notice if you're knock kneed—knees together, feet wide apart— when sitting or bending. This strains the outer hip and the inner knee. Avoid crossing the legs at the knees or pushing the hip out sideways while getting into a seat. Better to turn and face away from any seat we're sitting down on. This is especially true with car seats, a seat we often get into sideways. Sleeping with pillows between the knees helps to avoid the knock-kneed position when we're asleep.

Also, review the chapter on Balance and Walking (Chapter 8).

BUTTOCK STRETCH: STRONGER

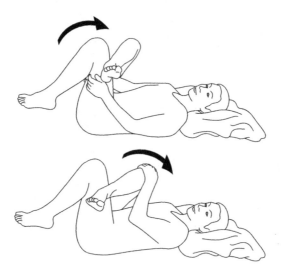

- Knees bent and feet flat on the bed or floor.
- Cross one ankle on other knee.
- Both hands grip thigh.
- Pull thigh toward chest lifting foot off bed (crossed knee is outward).
- Hold 3-5 seconds.
- Pull crossed knee inward toward opposite shoulder.
- Hold 3-5 seconds. Relax.
- Repeat 3-5 times.

BUTTOCK STRETCH: SITTING

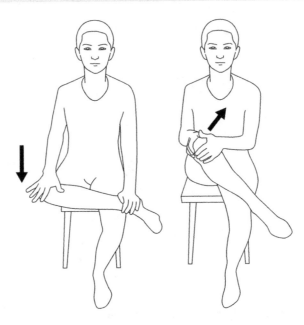

- Sit up straight on edge of chair.
- Cross one ankle on the other knee.
- Rock the pelvis forward like in PIL.
- Push the crossed knee toward the ground.
- As the knee is pushed downward, make an extra effort to rock the pelvis forward.
- Hold for 3-5 seconds.
- Pull the crossed knee up and in towards the opposite shoulder.
- Again, rock the pelvis forward.
- Hold 3-5 seconds. Relax.
- Repeat 3-5 times.
- Then, do the same on the other side. Notice if one side is easier to do than the other. That's often the case. If one side is stiffer, we know what we need to work on. Do this at least several times during the day.

BRIDGING

Bridging is a good way to strengthen hips and low back—in addition to using good body mechanics with bending and getting up from sitting.

Note: Do calf and hamstring stretches (pp. 194-196) before bridging to avoid muscle spasm.

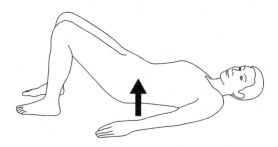

- Lie on the back with knees bent and feet flat about shoulder width apart. (This is actually easier to do on the floor or a firm surface than on a bed. Doing it on the bed will be more challenging.)
- Pull the belly in towards the spine, same as with PIL.
- Keep belly pulled in, lift the pelvis about 3-6 inches off the bed.
- Hold up to 10 seconds and lower slowly.
- Work up to 10 repetitions.

BRIDGING WITH MARCHING

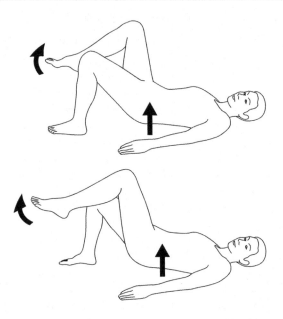

Make bridging more challenging:

- Bridge (lift hips), and keep pelvis level with the floor or bed.
- Lift up one leg at a time. Keep pelvis level.
- Move slowly, lifting alternate legs.
- Work up to 10 repetitions.
- This is great for strengthening and improving balance and coordination of the hips and trunk.

KNEES

Unlike hip pain, when knees are injured we feel pain around the knee joint and we know pretty well where the knee joint is. It could be in the front, the back, or the side of the joint, but we know it's the knee. Knees are the most unstable weight bearing joint in the body. That's why knee injuries, especially in sports, are so common. The knee joint is two long bones coming together—end on end—making a joint that's very vulnerable to sideways and twisting movements.

Knee Joint Anatomy

The knee is a joint with two parts. The weight-bearing part forms from the top of the tibia and the bottom of the femur—the tibiofemoral joint. The second, smaller joint is the kneecap—the patellofemoral joint. With injury or strain, swelling in either of these joints will prevent the knee from straightening all the way or bending completely.

There are four major ligaments that support the knee—on the inside (medial ligament), outside (lateral ligament), and two that cross deep in the middle of the joint (anterior and posterior cruciates). If you follow sports or have had a traumatic injury to your knee, you might be familiar with these names. In addition, there are two fibrous cushioning cartilages that are attached to the tibia (the shin bone). These are the "menisci" (Greek for crescent) named for their crescent shape. The quadriceps muscles—on the front of the thigh—cross over the front of the knee through the quadriceps tendon. The kneecap—patella—lies within the quadriceps tendon.

The quadriceps muscles (also known as "quads") straighten the knee. The hamstring muscles—on the back of the thigh—bend the knee. The longer calf muscle and the little, deep popliteus muscle also cross the joint in the back.

Tendons cross the inside and outside of the knee joint and help to stabilize it. When doing sports, or life in general, poor alignment of the knee makes side-to-side and twisting movements very risky. Learning good mechanics and muscular control of the knee, especially while training for sports, is the best defense against being injured. Simply put, knees work best when they bend over feet.

Subtle Knee Strains and Acute Care

We can strain either knee joint by an obvious, sudden twisting injury or more gradually from poor body mechanics. Knees can be strained by the way we run, the way we walk up stairs, or get out of a car or chair. Sitting with our feet hooked around a low rung on a chair or sitting with knees bent more than 90 degrees can strain the knees. Strain (stress on muscles) or sprain (stress on ligaments and menisci) is due to the angle of the bent knee, most commonly the knock kneed position, just like with hips.

A swollen knee joint is treated with RICE—Rest, Ice, Compression, and Elevation. Then we should make sure to do gentle exercise as soon as we're able. If we have a mild strain, slowly start getting the range of movement and strength back on the same day. Don't put off doing some exercise for more than 2-3 days. Do what you can. Use ice after doing gentle exercises.

Wearing an elastic support will help to control swelling and give a sense of stability of the joint. Take the elastic support off when doing these simple early rehab exercises and when using ice.

You will feel better, but not completely better, within 2-3 days if it's a minor strain/sprain. Call for medical advice if things aren't improving somewhat in 3-5 days, or if they aren't much better in 2-3 weeks.

FIRST THING TO DO FOR KNEE PAIN

- Bend and straighten knee without weight bearing—like slowly kicking a ball.
- Straighten knee fully and do a quad set (p. 192).
- In standing, do partial knee bends (pp. 198-199).
- Walk slowly with attention to foot contact on ground, knee bending over foot (pp. 84-85).

KNEE STRAIGHTENING

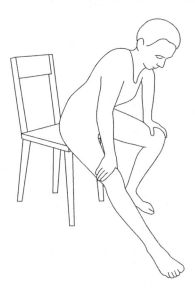

- Sit on the edge of a chair with the heel on the floor.
- If unable to straighten the knee fully, place one or both hands just above the knee on the lower part of the thigh above the kneecap. Don't push down on the kneecap.
- With the knee straightened as much as it can, push downward with the hands straightening it further. Don't push down towards the foot. Push perpendicular to the joint towards the floor. This may be felt in the back of the knee or in the front of the knee joint below the kneecap. This can be uncomfortable initially.
- Hold a few seconds and let the knee bend—sliding the foot back on the floor—to get relief and to let the blood flow around the knee. Movement is key to good blood flow and pain relief.
- Then straighten the knee again.
- Continue pushing the knee straight followed by bending.
- Repeat 3-5 times.

KNEE BENDING: EASIER

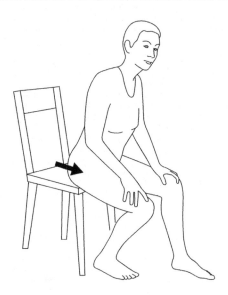

- With a very stiff knee, start by sitting deep in a chair with feet on floor.
- Keeping the foot on the floor, scoot hips forward, bending the knee further. (It's OK for the heel to lift up.)
- Hold 3-5 seconds. Relax.
- Straighten the knee and do a quad set (p. 192).
- Repeat bending and straightening 3-5 times.

KNEE BENDING: STRONGER

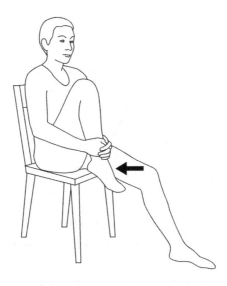

- When able to bend the knee more, lean back in the chair, lifting the thigh to bend the knee.
- Gently try to pull the ankle in toward the thigh. Use a towel looped around the ankle and pull the towel—if reaching with hands is difficult.
- Hold 3-5 seconds.
- Always follow the bending of the knee with straightening and doing a quad set (p. 192).
- Repeat 3-5 times.

KNEE STRENGTHENING: QUAD SETS

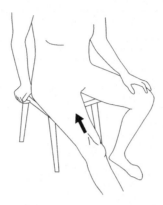

A "quad set" is tightening the front of the thigh with the knee fully straightened. You want to be able to lift the leg off the floor keeping the knee straight.

This strength in the knee is key to solving many knee joint problems. We always need to start with these exercises to hasten the recovery from knee injury or after surgery.

- With the knee straight, tighten the quad muscles on the front of the thigh.
- If unable to straighten the knee completely, do a quad set with the knee as straight as possible.
- Hold 3-5 seconds. Relax.
- Repeat 3-5 times.

Note: Quad sets are good to do as needed, in bed or standing with the knee straight, until they become pain free.

KNEE STRENGTHENING: STRAIGHT LEG RAISE

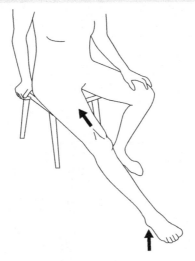

- With the quad muscles tightened, keep the knee straight and lift the heel slightly off the floor. This is a "straight leg raise."
- Hold for 5-10 seconds, doing 5-10 repetitions.
- Relax and repeat 1-3 times.
- Once you can do the quad set and straight leg raise well, then do a straight leg raise with the hip turned outward—toes pointing outward. This helps to strengthen the inner part of the quad and inner thigh, which helps the kneecap to move well.

Difficulty Doing Straight Leg Raise

If unable to do a straight leg raise without the knee bending, the quad is weak. Try doing it in standing—it takes less strength in standing. Continue to work on tightening the front of the thigh—doing quad sets. Continue to do quad sets, every hour or more, until you're able to lift the leg keeping the knee straight.

Quad sets and basic straight leg raises without knee pain are key to a healthy, happy knee. If painful at first, like always, do it slowly. Hold a few seconds and relax. Then try it again, and go back and forth a few times, tightening the thigh and relaxing, until it can be tightened without pain. This could take a little time, so keep working on it throughout the day.

GASTROCNEMIUS STRETCH: SUPERFICIAL CALF

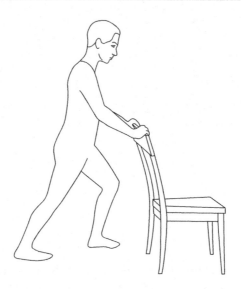

- Hold onto something for balance.
- Feet shoulder width apart, take a big step back with one leg.
- Feet pointing forward, weight on outer border of the feet, toes in contact with floor.
- Keep the back knee as straight as possible and bend the front knee, keeping the back heel on the floor.
- Feel a stretch in the back of the leg and knee.
- Hold 5-10 seconds. Relax.
- Repeat 2-3 times if a strong stretch is felt.

SOLEUS STRETCH: DEEP CALF

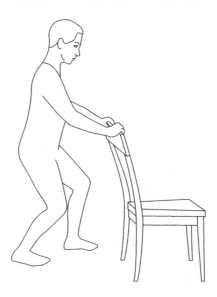

- Take a shorter step back to do this stretch. The toes of the back foot are even with the heel of the front foot.
- Feet are pointing forward, weight on outer border of feet, toes in contact with the floor.
- Bend both knees.
- Hold 5-10 seconds. Relax.
- Repeat 2-3 times if a strong stretch is felt.

HAMSTRING STRETCH: BACK OF THIGH

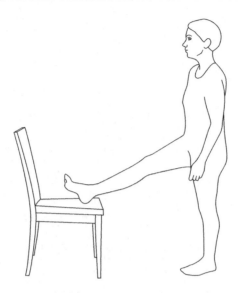

- Stand facing a chair. Hold onto something for balance if needed.
- Lift the heel onto the seat of the chair with the knee straight. If the chair seat is too high, have the heel on something lower, like a step.
- Standing leg and pelvis are straight, facing the leg being stretched.
- Stand tall, rocking the pelvis forward like in PIL.
- Feel the stretch in the back of the thigh. If not feeling much stretch, maintain forward pelvic position and bend forward in the hip with the chest up.
- Roll the leg on the chair in and out slowly, alternating toes pointing inward, toes pointing outward.
- Continue for 5-10 seconds, rolling the leg in and out.

QUADRICEPS STRETCH: FRONT OF THIGH

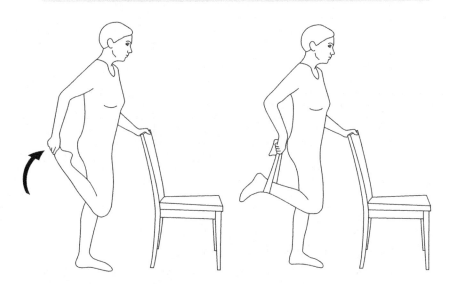

- Hold onto something for balance if needed.
- To control the stretch use a towel or strap around the ankle. If we can grab the ankle to do the stretch, that's fine.
- After grabbing the ankle—one way or another— pull the heel in towards the buttocks and straighten the hip, trying to keep the knee pointing downwards and the pelvis level.
- For the final part, just like with the hip flexor muscle, rock the pelvis backward, flattening the low back. A pull is felt in front of the thigh and knee.
- Pull the heel towards the buttock 3-5 seconds.
- Relax, straightening the knee.
- Pull again 3-5 times.

DOUBLE LEG KNEE BENDS AND HEEL RAISES

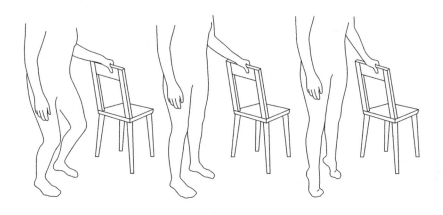

- Stand with the feet shoulder width apart.
- Bend the knees slightly, knees over the toes but not past them. (Bending the knees past the toes causes excessive pressure on the kneecaps.) Knees are open and weight is on the outer border of the feet with the toes in contact with the floor.
- Straighten the knees and do a quad set.
- Keep the knees straight and lift the heels off floor. Weight is on the big toes.
- Lower the heels, with the knees straight. Relax quads.
- Repeat knee bend, knee straightening and heel raise.
- Do slowly, 5-10 times.

Note: Review Standing Up and Sitting Down (p. 66) and Chair Squats (p. 67) for the correct mechanics of knee bending. Chair squats are good to do after knee bends become easy.

SINGLE LEG KNEE BEND AND HEEL RAISE

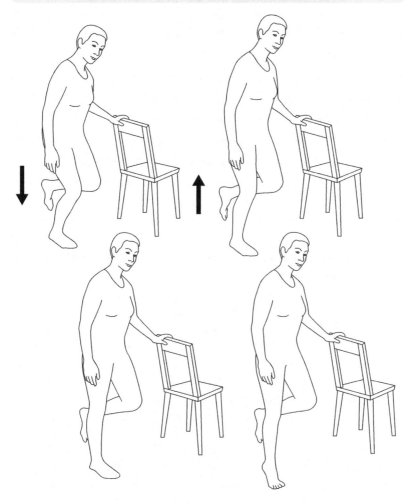

- Progress to single leg knee bend by putting slightly more weight on the injured leg until it's able to bear all the weight. For support, initially hold onto a counter.
- Bend the knee slightly, knee over toes.
- Straighten the knee. Do a quad set.
- Keep the knee straight. Lift the heel off floor. Weight on the big toe.
- Lower the heel.
- Repeat 5-10 times.

PRACTICE JUMPING

Note: Only do this if jumping is a part of your life that you want to get back to.

- Stand with hands on a counter.
- Do partial knee bend with both legs and straighten the knees.
- As you do the heel raise, push down with hands to support weight and lift the feet off floor pointing the toes.
- Return to floor with the toes first, bending the knees as heels touch the floor, and then go into a deeper knee bend.
- Practice jumping with good mechanics away from the counter.

Knee Joint Hyperextension: Hypermobility and Bad Habits

Some people are hypermobile and have very flexible joints. This is often most evident in the knee joint. Knees are not just straight, but bow backwards. This is hyperextension of the knee and it's not good to let it go unchecked. It makes the knee more vulnerable to injury by weakening the quadriceps and having less control of the joint.

Even if we're not hypermobile in other joints, some people habitually fully extend the knees—straightening to the end of range—when walking, standing, or playing sports. They land hard on a straight knee, instead of lightly on a slightly bent knee.

Once we become aware of this habit, stop doing it! Like any change in habit, we'll have to walk slower to practice our new way of walking and be conscious of how we're standing. It's important to be able to fully straighten the knee and to be able to lift the leg with the knee locked straight. But we don't want to be forcefully bearing weight with the knee completely straight as we walk or land from jumping. As we're landing on the leg with walking, running, or jumping, we need all the muscles around the knee to be controlling the knee. This provides stability. Weight-bearing on a fully straightened knee relies on the stability of the joint itself, and the knee joint doesn't have that much stability to offer.

STRENGTHENING KNEES AND HIPS ON STAIRS

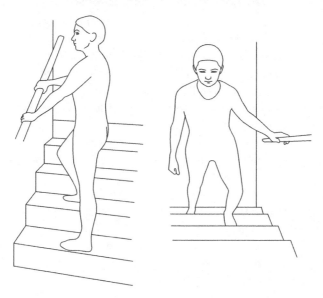

Often it's very difficult, or impossible, to walk up stairs normally after a knee injury or surgery. Walking up stairs sideways is less painful and a good way to strengthen the knee and hip.

- Face sideways toward stair railing, both hands on railing.
- Step up sideways with the weaker leg, keeping the knee open and the foot facing towards the railing.
- Before stepping up, do PIL.
- Then step up slowly.
- Continue up a few stairs and then come back down stairs slowly.
- When beginning to walk up stairs normally, make sure to have the knee open and the foot straight ahead.

The Overlooked Popliteus Muscle

I saw a lot of knee injuries when I was working in the clinic and I have had a lot of knee injuries myself. I became an expert knee clinician when I realized how important a certain short muscle behind the knee is. The popliteus muscle is deep within the back of the knee joint—one of those important deep muscles again. It initiates a rotational movement of normal knee mechanics. It has attachments to the outer, lateral meniscus—the cushioning cartilage of the knee. Apparently many therapists and doctors forget about the poor little popliteus, but if you remember it, you become "an expert," too!

I had my own popliteus go into spasm by riding up a steep hill on my mountain bike without warming up. If the popliteus goes into spasm, it can feel like a torn meniscus since the muscle attaches to this cartilage. Having also had a torn meniscal carti-lage, I know how both injuries feel. They feel exactly the same! The knee gets stuck or caught. You can bend it, but not straight-en it fully. This is often described as being "locked". (Not to be confused with a quad set "locked" knee.) If we have a locked knee from a torn meniscus, the torn cartilage blocks the knee joint from straightening. But if we haven't had any trauma to the knee, what feels like a torn cartilage might just be the popliteus muscle in spasm, preventing the knee from straightening. Take the time to push and straighten the knee gently. (This is also OK to try if you have a torn meniscus. You just might not make any headway.) Doing this stretches the popliteus. Bending and then straightening the knee back and forth, gently gets the muscle out of spasm and it stops pulling on that lateral meniscus. We might have to do this throughout the day until the muscle is out of spasm. Another good reason to occasionally do knee straightening and quad sets!

ANKLES, FEET, TOES

My first injury as a kid was a sprained ankle. I found the whole thing fascinating. The swelling of the joint and use of ice was interesting. Wrapping the ankle with an ace bandage and hobbling around was kind of different. Mostly I was just hanging around the house for a few days and reading an Amelia Earhart biography and watching TV. Not so bad.

Of the recovery, I have no recollection. I was an active kid and soft tissues are much more fluid and pliable when we're younger. It just got better.

Spraining my ankle in my late 40s was a different story. It turned all blue from the partial tearing of ligaments. I did the RICE (Rest, Ice, Compression, Elevation) treatment with one difference: I started moving my ankle up and down slightly the same day I sprained it. Holding my leg up in the air to let gravity help reduce the swelling, I worked my calf muscles as best I could. I had a James Brown concert to go to in a couple of days. I had to get back to work and go see James Brown! Motivation was high. Using a cane at first, I walked slowly without limping. Wearing an elastic support, I went to the concert, and less memorably, was back to work walking slowly without a cane after a few days. I progressed completely in 2 weeks by doing all the ankle exercises below.

So here's the deal: Moving a joint slowly, soon after an injury, is a good thing. Unless a bone is broken, then it's a bad thing. Don't push it hard; just do small movements a few times, a few times a day. It speeds up the whole process. Like with the knee, wear an elastic support to help control swelling and give a feeling of better stability while the ankle heals.

FIRST THING TO DO FOR ANKLE/FOOT PAIN

- Do ankle/foot movements below.
- In standing, do partial knee bends (pp.198-199).
- Walk slowly with attention to foot contact on ground (pp. 84-85).

ANKLE MOVEMENT IN SITTING OR STANDING

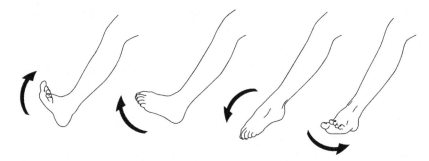

- Move the foot and ankle around, up and down, and in a circle.
- Pull the toes up as the foot comes up and point the toes down as the foot goes down. Make these movements as big as possible.
- Then, repeat the stretch with the heel on the floor, scooting forward in the chair several times (p. 204).
- For a stronger stretch, cross the ankle on the knee and use the hands to pull and push the ankle and foot back and forth, and in a circle slowly. Then move ankle in a circle (as above).
- Repeat 3-5 times.

ANKLE STRETCH: EASIER

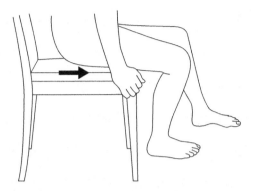

- Sit deep in a chair with the foot flat on the floor.
- Keeping the heel on the floor, scoot forward in the chair. This is felt in the front of the ankle. If unable to do this with the heel on the floor, let it come off the floor slightly.
- Then, repeat the stretch with the heel on the floor.
- Hold 5-10 seconds and relax, doing ankle movements below.
- Repeat 3-5 times.

Cautionary Tale

If we haven't done calf and ankle stretches after a broken or sprained ankle, we start walking again no matter what. That stiff ankle will just get better by walking around. Right? Well, that can be true, but it depends on how we walk. If we haven't gotten back our flexibility in the ankle and foot, we'll propel ourselves forward as best we can. The lack of flexibility will make the foot turn outward. As the foot turns outward we push off the side of the big toe, not straight over it. The knee starts bending over the arch of the stiff foot and ankle, not over the toes. We start to get foot pain in the heel and arch, bunions on the big toe, and often knee pain on the inside of the knee. Then we think "Oh great, now my whole foot and knee hurt. Where did I put those pain pills?"

But don't despair. Even if we've been walking like this for way too long, we can still bounce back by changing the mechanics of walking (Chapter 8) by taking shorter steps and by doing the stretches described here.

ANKLE STRETCHES IN STANDING

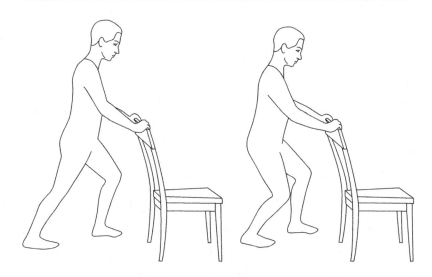

- With a stiff ankle you will feel pressure in the front of the ankle with calf stretches.
- Start with the gastrocnemius stretch with the back knee straight.
- Then do the soleus stretch with the back knee bent.
- As the joint becomes more mobile, feel a stretch in the back of the leg and knee.
- Hold 5-10 seconds. Relax and do the ankle movements above.
- Repeat 3-5 times.

TOE STRETCHES: TOES UP

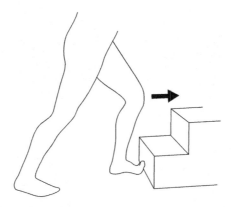

- To stretch the toes, find a step and put the toes on the step riser. (This is best to do barefoot, or with flexible shoes.)
- Keeping the heel down, bend the knee.
- Hold 5-10 seconds. Relax.
- Repeat 3-5 times.

Note: This is great for plantar fasciitis, bunion prevention, or for any heel or arch pain. Review Walking Basics (p. 84).

TOE STRETCHES: TOES DOWN

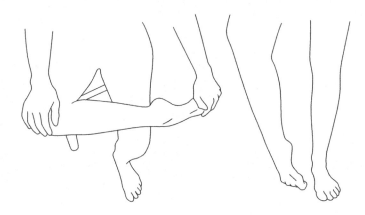

- In sitting, cross the ankle on the knee.
- Pull the foot and toes in and upward towards the big toe.
- In standing, point the foot downward like a ballerina.
- Rest the top of the toes (the toe nail side) on the floor and push the ankle forward.
- With the toes pointed inward and the heel outward, stretch the front of the shin.
- Hold 3-5 seconds.
- Repeat 3-5 times.

Note: This is good for pain along the shin (shin splints) and a good stretch for the front of the ankle.

Plantar Fasciitis and Stretching Feet in Bed

Plantar fasciitis is a common problem that causes foot pain. The plantar fascia is a tough connective tissue that extends from the heel to the ball of the foot— at the base of the big toe to the pinky toe. It helps to support the arch in the foot. This tissue can get inflamed and irritated by all the abuse we can do to the feet. Feet will really let us know what they don't like! Maybe it was that new pair of shoes that gave no support while we walked miles on concrete. Or was it using a shovel while wearing shoes with flimsy soles. Then every time we get out of bed or stand up from a chair, we get that pain message. Ow!

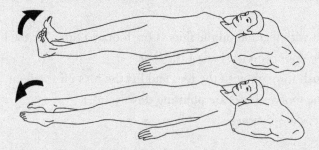

It's important to stretch the feet and toes while we're still in bed. As we sleep, the feet are pointing downwards. When we have foot pain, we need to stretch before we get out of bed and walk.

- Pull the toes and ankles up first. To avoid getting a nasty cramp, a charley horse in the calf, it's better not to point the feet downward first.
- Do it a few times until there's no pain. Lying on the back we can even let the bed covers help to give us a stretch. Hold 3-5 seconds.
- Then point the toes and ankles downward. Hold 1-2 seconds.
- Pull the toes and ankles up and down 3-5 times or until movement is pain free—or with minimal pain.

SITTING HEEL LIFTS

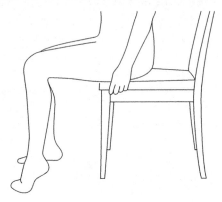

- Sit with feet flat on the floor: One foot at a time, lift the heel off the floor onto the ball of the foot.
- Push through with the toes and lift the toes off the floor.
- The foot and toes are pointing downward.
- Repeat 3-5 times.

SITTING FOOT AND TOE RAISES

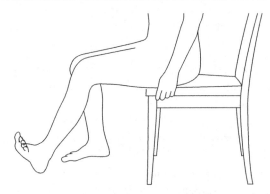

- Sit with feet flat on the floor. Keeping the heels on the floor, lift the toes and feet.
- With the heels down and the toes and feet up, move the feet outward towards the little toes and inward towards the big toes.
- Keep the knees still to avoid hip movement.

STRENGTHENING ANKLES AND FEET

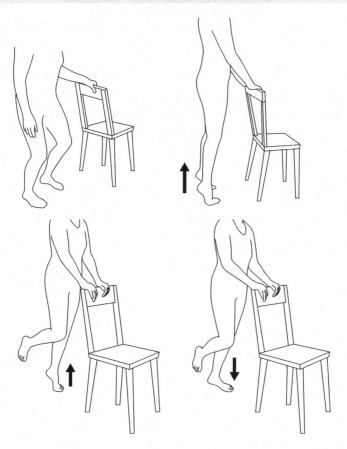

Note: Refer to Double and Single Leg Knee Bends and Heel Raises in Knee section above.

To progress to single leg toe raise after a foot or ankle injury:

- Hold on for support. Begin standing on both legs.
- Raise the heels.
- Shift more weight onto the injured foot and lower the heels.
- Repeat 5-10 times.
- Gradually progress to going up on two feet and down on one, 5 -10 times.
- Then progress to up and down on one foot, 5-10 times.

Ankle Sprains Versus Fractures

Typically we "sprain" the outer ankle ligaments if the foot rolls inward. We "break" the ankle if the foot rolls outward. To be clear, a break is the same as a fracture. Sometimes with a very forceful sprain we can have an "avulsion fracture." That's when a piece of bone is pulled away by a ligament or tendon. An X-ray is recommended after a high impact trauma, especially if unable to bear any weight—even painfully—on the leg. Immobilization is required for an avulsion fracture of the joint.

With a worse, even more forceful injury, bones can be fractured. Typically, fractures can involve the lower part of the tibia—long bone on the inside of the leg—and the lower part of the fibula—long bone on the outside of the leg.

Coming out of a cast after having a broken ankle or surgery for a broken ankle is a little different than working with a sprained ankle. The ankle is incredibly stiff after it's been completely immobilized in a cast while the bone is healing, 4-8 weeks. (It also needs a good washing and some cream applied to it. The skin looks and smells icky.) Full recovery can take 2-6 months or longer. So we have to push harder to get it moving. To speed things up, its great if we can see a PT to help us get going in the right direction.

In both cases, whether stretching an ankle after a break or after a sprain, using ice after stretching will feel good. A really stiff ankle that's healed feels better with heat before doing the stretches. We can always use ice afterwards. If we have persistent swelling after the injury, use an elastic ankle support. We want to be up and moving but we need to control swelling. When sitting, elevate the leg to prevent more swelling. Best to recline to avoid over-stretching the hamstring muscles and pulling the sciatic nerve.

Reminder

Review Chapter 7 and Chapter 8 to put everything "From the Ground Up" together. Getting the foot and knee alignment right (knee bending over the foot), the hip will follow. Functional strength—everyday movement using good alignment and mechanics—is what excellent self-care of the hips, knees, ankles, and feet is all about.

Chapter 15

The Body Electric
Nerve Problems

A woman who worked in a busy office was referred to physical
therapy for a wrist strain. She had gotten sick and had to cancel
her original appointment. While she wasn't at work, a younger person had been hired and she feared losing her job. Feeling better after
having rested for a few days, she worked with a vengeance on her
backlog of work. Further stress at work started to give her neck pain.

A few days later her wrist pain came back, but much worse
than before. Burning, tingling pain started traveling up her arm
and into her shoulder. The pain was excruciating. She started using
her other arm for the mouse on her computer and held her painful
arm across her chest.

She went back to her doctor who took an X-ray of her neck,
which showed degenerative changes of osteoarthritis and disc degen-
eration. This caused even more concern for her. The pain intensified.
The doctor again suggested she go to physical therapy. She used the
original prescription she was given for a wrist strain.

215

*I double-checked her referral when she walked through the door
to make sure I was seeing the right patient. I would have guessed by
the way she held her arm across her chest, that she had experienced
a stroke. (A stroke is an injury to the brain where the blood supply
has been altered, often leaving a person unable to use an extremity.) Because of pain, this woman had completely disabled herself by
not using her arm for weeks. She hadn't had a stroke, but she had a
condition called "adverse mechanical neural tension," resulting in
nerve pain that limits mobility. Due to the sensitivity of her nervous system—in this case, the nerves from her neck that travel into
her arm—any movement of her arm was unbearable.*

*This woman did improve with PT treatment and seeing a psy-
chotherapist for stress management counseling. After a few months
she was able to use her arm normally again. This is a good example
of how thoughts can affect the body. Or what happens if we are unaware of the signs of adverse mechanical neural tension and, more
likely, have never heard of it before! Our bodies can get our attention in most unpleasant ways.*

Most of us have seen bones and muscles. We can see examples in
the grocery store meat department. But how many of us have seen a
nervous system? In 1925 two medical students took over 1000 hours to
dissect the body's peripheral nervous system, including the spinal cord,
keeping it in a continuous piece. No easy task. It looks like a feathery,
branching, strange tree with the legs being the roots, the spinal cord
the trunk, and the head and arms the branches.

Unlike bones and muscles that start and stop, the nervous system
is a continuous tissue that includes the brain and spinal cord and all
the nerves that run to the head, trunk, arms, legs, and internal organs.
Nerves send electric messages from the brain throughout the body and
vice versa along the same nerve fibers. Nerve tissue itself is very strong.
You can pull hard on a nerve and it won't tear. Nerves are tolerant of
fast movement—think of a gymnast or most any sport movements—as
well as being relatively still while sleeping.

Nerves are most sensitive to lack of blood flow. If you've ever fallen asleep with your arm hanging off the edge of the bed, or leaned on your arm for too long, it becomes painfully numb until we move and shake it back to life. In a less dramatic way, nerves create abnormal numbness, tingling, or pain if we've been in a stressful position for too long, such as sitting at a desk or driving and not moving enough. We can also have these symptoms if there's pressure on a nerve from a muscle spasm or soft tissue swelling from trauma. Nerves can often tolerate slow progressive pressures of degenerative spinal conditions. Degenerative conditions develop slowly over time. This can explain why bad looking X-rays don't necessarily correspond to painful symptoms (Chapter 4).

So what are nerve symptoms? They can be numbness, tingling, burning sensation, pain, or other weird sensations like a feeling of water trickling on the skin.

When nerve symptoms become more severe they can also cause weakness in an extremity, like having a foot drop with a sciatic nerve problem in the leg. We're unable to lift the foot, allowing the heel to hit the ground first when taking a step. Instead, the foot slaps on the ground without control. If we have an onset of weakness—not due to pain—in the arms or legs, we need to seek medical attention immediately.

But like everything, an ounce of prevention is worth a pound of cure. Doing PIL frequently during the day is the best way to avoid having these symptoms and to begin recovery from trauma. PIL relieves stress to the entire continuous peripheral nervous system.

ULNAR NERVE: THE "FUNNY" BONE

A nerve in the arm that we might all be familiar with is "the funny bone." Apparently, some people think sharp stabbing nerve pain is funny. When we hit the inner edge of the elbow just right we get a most unpleasant electric sensation. Yes, it is the humerus bone, but still, it's not funny.

The ulnar nerve is very superficial as it crosses the elbow at the point where it can get hit. In fact, the ulnar nerve is the least protected nerve in our body. It's also very superficial as it crosses the palm side of our wrist toward the little finger. When tweaked or hit, this nerve pain can be felt on the little finger side of the forearm, into the little finger and ring finger.

I saw a man once who had the ultimate funny bone injury. As he slipped going down stairs, his elbow somehow smashed into a drinking glass, breaking it. The nerve was injured and had been surgically repaired. The only way he could be comfortable was to have his elbow and wrist straight with his arm turned inward, palm outward, and thumb pointing down. This is the position with the least amount of pull on the ulnar nerve.

Short of having that kind of injury, we can irritate this nerve by bending or leaning on the elbow for too long without moving. Some of us have the habit of sleeping with elbows and wrists bent up and hands tucked under the chin or cheek. This is a great way for us to get this nerve annoyed.

MEDIAN NERVE: CARPAL TUNNEL

Another nerve in the arm that is easily irritated is the median nerve. This nerve runs through the carpal tunnel. The carpal tunnel is a very narrow, confined space on the palm side of the wrist joint. It's filled with blood vessels and tendons that can get inflamed and swollen. Median nerve pain is often called carpal tunnel syndrome. Pain is felt in the palm side of the wrist, into the palm side of the thumb and index finger, sometimes the middle finger. If we work or sleep with the wrist bent, pressure—from swelling or compression—can build in this tight space. Nerves hate prolonged pressures and lack of blood flow.

RADIAL NERVE: TENNIS ELBOW

The radial nerve is the other major nerve in the arm and hand. It runs on the backside of the forearm and hand, which is where symptoms are felt. This nerve can get irritated after a prolonged strain to the forearm muscle, which pulls up the back of the hand. It can begin with tennis elbow. Problems often begin with a strained muscle and then develop into nerve pain.

CERVICAL RADICULOPATHY

This is nerve pain originating in the neck. Most commonly, you know if you have a cervical radiculopathy if you feel pain into the arm when you turn the head to the side, look up arching the neck backward, or bending the neck forward. These movements are to be avoided while the nerve is irritated and causing pain into the arm. At the same time, PIL is important to do faithfully, and perhaps obsessively, until the pain resolves. To check to see if pain is getting better, it's OK to slowly turn the head. But stop with the first onset of arm pain. Just once is enough!

SCIATIC NERVE: SCIATICA (LUMBAR RADICULOPATHY)

Many of us are personally familiar with the sciatic nerve. It even has a syndrome named after it: Sciatica. This is a general term that describes a nerve pain or tingling felt in the leg coming from an injury or strain to the low back or somewhere along the course of the nerve.

The sciatic nerve is the longest nerve in the body. If we've ever suffered with this condition, we know the anatomy fairly well. This nerve runs from the low back into the buttock, down the back of the thigh, into the back and side of the leg, and into the foot. It can be felt in some of these spots but not all. It's possible to just have foot pain that's sciatic.

Symptoms can be worse after doing anything that puts excessive static stretch or pull on this long nerve. It's pulled when we're sitting in a low seat with legs up and knees straight, or sitting slumped as we drive with one leg on the accelerator. (Review Chapter 7, Body Mechanics; and Chapter 9, Chairs and Beds.) It's a good guess that pain in the leg is from the sciatic nerve if we can get rid of it by doing the PIL position while standing and walking slowly.

FEMORAL NERVE: NERVE ENTRAPMENT

Sometimes when people hear the word "femoral" they think they've heard "ephemeral." We can only wish that any nerve pain would be ephemeral.

Named for the thigh's femur bone, the femoral nerve travels down the front of the thigh. Sometimes mechanical problems interfere with this nerve, such as tight fitting pants that pinch off the groin. A body type with a heavy abdomen and thighs and tight skin across the groin, tight hip flexor muscles, or trauma to the pelvis can also cause problems with this nerve. Numbness, tingling, or pain is felt in the groin, the front and outer side of the thigh and front of the knee.

FIRST THING TO DO FOR NERVE SYMPTOMS

- Stand and do PIL.
- For arm symptoms, emphasize palms forward, shoulder blades pinched together, lengthening the back of the neck. Hold a few seconds. Relax. Repeat 3-5 times.
- For leg symptoms, emphasize lengthening the spine and pulling the belly in towards the spine.
- Walk slowly doing PIL.

Radiculopathy

Nerves branch off from the spinal cord. Nerve roots are the part of the nerves that exit between the vertebrae of the spine. A radiculopathy is literally an irritation or injury to the nerve root, "radix" meaning "root" in Latin. A cervical radiculopathy is a problem coming from the neck; a lumbosacral radiculopathy is a problem coming from the low back. Pressure on these nerves can be from a spasm in the muscles between the vertebrae or some kind of swelling in that area. It could also indicate degenerative boney changes coupled with poor postural and body mechanic habits. The ulnar, median, and radial nerves all branch off from nerves coming from nerve roots in the neck. The sciatic and femoral nerves branch off from nerve roots from the lumbosacral spine.

Nerves need blood flow and movement to improve, not prolonged stretching. Always keep moving slowly when you do these exercises. Never hold these positions. Move slowly—as always—and stop at onset of increased symptoms. That's far enough to go. Do a few repetitions and then return to PIL. While symptoms might be felt a little stronger when you first do them, a minute after stopping, they should feel better. If this isn't the case, then the movement was too strong. Do a more gentle repetition or stick with PIL and try again the next day.

ULNAR AND MEDIAN NERVE MOBILIZATION: EASIER

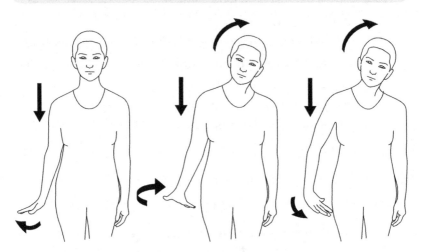

- Standing or sitting: Begin with PIL with the arm at the side.
- On the problem side, shrug the shoulder up.
- Relax.
- To continue, stand erect, but not actively doing PIL.
- Pull the hand back so the palm and fingers are facing the floor.
- Remain standing straight—no side-bending—and press down with the arm as if trying to touch the palm to the floor.
- Then relax. If symptoms are not aggravated, press down again trying to touch the palm to the floor and tilt the head away from that side.
- Then relax. If still OK—slight increase in pulling or tingling but not worse pain—press down with the arm, tilt the head away from the painful side, and rotate the arm in so fingers are pointing to the thigh. Then rotate the arm so the fingers point away from the body and then backwards. Feel a slight pull, maybe a little tingling, keep moving a few times, rotating the arm in and out.
- Relax.

ULNAR AND MEDIAN NERVE MOBILIZATION: STRONGER

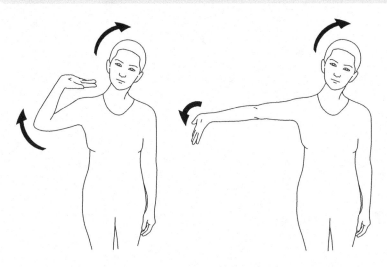

Note: Remember to keep moving in and out of these positions slowly.

- Press the shoulder down, palm facing the floor, tilting the head away, as fingers are pointing in towards the thigh.
- Bend the elbow and raise the forearm so fingertips are pointing towards the neck.
- The final move: Straighten the elbow so the arm is away from the body, fingers pointing downward.
- Again bend the elbow, fingers pointing to neck.
- Straighten the elbow, fingers pointing downward.
- Bend and straighten the elbow a few times.
- Relax with the arm at the side.

RADIAL NERVE MOBILIZATION

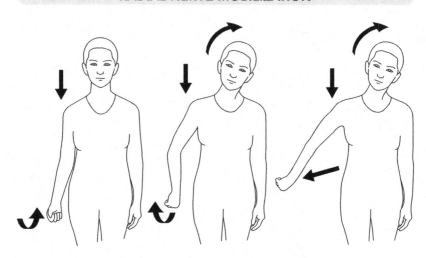

- Standing or sitting: Do PIL with the arm at the side.
- Make a fist with the thumb into palm and fingers wrapped around the thumb.
- Pull the wrist back, palm towards the forearm.
- Press the shoulder down, tilt head away from the painful side.
- Rotate the arm, turning with the thumb facing backward. The palm is facing outward.
- Bend the elbow and then straighten it.
- Keep moving the elbow back and forth a few times and then relax.

SCIATIC NERVE MOBILIZATION: EASIER

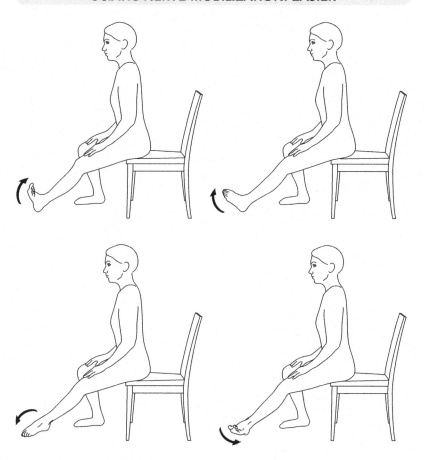

- Sit at the edge of the chair, leg out straight, heel on the floor with knee straight.
- Do PIL.
- Pull the toes and foot up. Point the toes and foot down.
- Repeat 3-5 times.
- Rotate the toes and foot in a circle.
- Repeat 3-5 times.
- Walk taking short steps while doing PIL for 30-60 seconds.

SCIATIC NERVE MOBILIZATION: STRONGER - SITTING

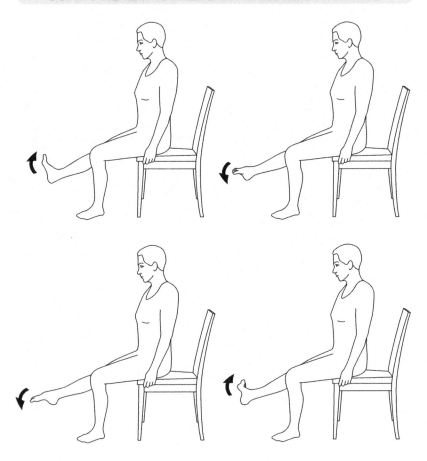

- Sit at the edge of the chair.
- Do PIL.
- Lift the leg off floor slightly with knee straight.
- Rotate the foot and toes in a circle and up and down a few times.
- Stand up from the chair doing PIL with good body mechanics.
- Walk taking short steps while doing PIL for 30-60 seconds.

SCIATIC NERVE MOBILIZATION: STRONGER - STANDING

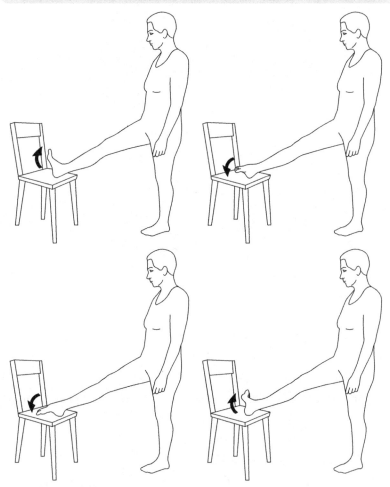

- Hold on for balance if needed.
- Facing the chair, place the heel on the seat.
- Do PIL.
- Pull toes and foot up, then point the toes and foot down.
- Repeat 3-5 times.
- Rotate the toes and foot in a circle.
- Repeat 3-5 times.
- Put the foot back on the ground. Walk taking short steps while doing PIL for 30-60 seconds.

FEMORAL NERVE MOBILIZATION

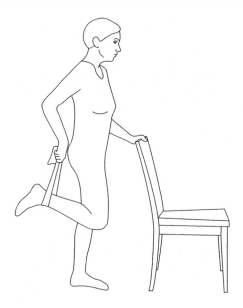

- Get a long towel or strap.
- Hold on for balance.
- Loop the towel or strap around the front of the ankle. Hold the other ends with a hand on the same side as the leg being mobilized.
- Tuck the pelvis under—flattening the back. This is opposite of the pelvic position with PIL.
- Bending the elbow, pull the towel/strap upward, bending the knee as far as comfortable. The knee is pointing towards the floor.
- Straighten the elbow, allowing the knee to partially straighten.
- Bend and straighten the knee.
- Repeat 3-5 times.
- Walk taking short steps while doing PIL for 30-60 seconds.

Fine Tuning Neural Mobilization

At each progressive step of neural mobilization exercises we want to ask ourselves if the symptoms are feeling worse and getting stronger.

We want to move to the point of having a slight increase in symptoms. As symptoms improve, we can progress further.

Do neural mobilization exercises on only one arm or leg at a time. Why? The nervous system is all connected. Unlike muscles and tendons that go from one point to another, nerves come from the brain and spine and go everywhere. Moving both arms or legs at the same time creates a very strong pull to sensitive nerves. If we're not having any problems, it doesn't matter much. But if we're having some kind of nerve pain, or if we're checking to see if the symptom involves a nerve in one arm or leg, we want to move one limb at a time.

If having nerve symptoms, continue to do PIL frequently during the day and do neural mobilization exercises, a few repetitions, as needed throughout the day. Symptoms should improve, at least temporarily, within a minute of doing the exercises. Catching and treating symptoms early, complete and lasting improvement can happen within minutes. Avoid any prolonged stretches while still having symptoms. Mobilization means movement.

Easiest, Best Neural Mobilization Exercise: Walking

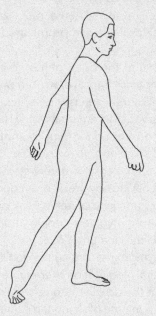

Now it's time to recognize that there's something we've been doing all our lives that's really great for the health of the nerves in the arms and legs, not to mention our health in general. Walking! Opposite arms and legs swinging along is just what nerves love. The heart is pumping, blood is flowing, lungs are expanding, breathing is deeper, muscles are contracting and relaxing, and nerves are getting that back and forth movement that they love.

It's best to start walking slowly, doing PIL as we walk, exaggerating the arm swing—but as we warm up, we can move a little faster. If we're having nerve pain, best to walk on level surfaces until we start feeling better.

Reminder

Nerve pain or other nerve symptoms don't have to be a mystery anymore. Learn these exercises so it's easy to use them wherever and whenever they're needed. And once again—always start with PIL!

SUMMARY OF PART FOUR

1. Joints depend on movement for the health of soft tissue deep in joints (synovium) and the surrounding soft tissue (bursa). With swelling, full range of motion of joints is limited. It's important to regain full movement of joints for good self-care.

2. Soft tissue injury is repaired by collagen fibers. Progressive stretching and strengthening helps to organize collagen fibers after injury to tolerate normal stresses. This is key to recovery and good function of healing soft tissue.

3. A few repetitions of joint movements as needed during daily activities should be done until full range of motion is restored and pain relieved. This may take a few repetitions if caught early, or days or weeks if having a more severe or chronic condition. Continue to work on areas where mobility and strength are a problem.

4. For any neck, mid back, low back, shoulder, jaw, or hip pain, first do PIL in standing or sitting.

5. When having a problem with one joint, it's a good idea to do the movements for surrounding joints at least once to check for possible related mobility problems. Examples: For elbow pain, do elbow, shoulder, and wrist/hand exercises; for shoulder pain, do shoulder, neck and elbow exercise; for knee pain, do knee, hip and ankle exercises; for low back pain do hip and mid back exercises; for neck pain, do shoulder and mid back exercises.

6. After any injury or strain, do neural mobilization exercises briefly to check the tolerance of nerve mobility.

7. First do PIL and then do neural mobilization exercises (slow, continuous movement) for any numbness, tingling, or other weird sensations in the arms or legs.

Epilogue

What? No Magical Fix?
You Are More Powerful Than You Know

*W*orking as a manual physical therapist, I developed the skills needed to treat orthopedic problems by using hands-on techniques. There are times when results can be dramatic. Suddenly a person is able to turn their neck without pain. Right after treatment, the backache is gone and full movement is restored. More often, manual treatments—for mild to moderate injuries—require several visits and follow through with exercises and instructions.

The goal is to maintain improvement and prevent relapse. But if symptoms return, many people only remember the "magic" of the manual treatment and not the self-care instructions. "She did something to me that made me feel better and I need to go in for another treatment!"

Early in my career I was seeing a woman for shoulder, neck, and low back pain. She had a young family and worked a full-time office job with a 5 hour round trip commute. Lots of sitting! Finally, with *increasing discomfort and being unable to sleep, she made time to come in for physical therapy. Returning for her second appointment, she let me know that her pain had only temporarily changed after the manual therapy treatment. She hadn't done any of the exercises I'd prescribed because she didn't have time to do them.*

I remember thinking, and I hope I didn't say it out loud, "Well, of course you're in pain! You don't have any time for yourself and your life is incredibly stressful!" I observed my emotional reaction to her and thought, "Wait a minute. This is her life. It's not going to change. I'm the one who needs to change." With that epiphany I improved my approach and began to give her movements and strengthening exercises she could do during her commute, at work at her desk, in bed before she slept, and when she first woke up. This helped me realize that for everyone—busy or not—self-care has to fit into daily life. That's the only way it really makes sense. I might see someone for 30 minutes once every week, but they are with themselves all the rest of the time! What people do—and learn to do—for themselves is much more significant than what manual skills alone can do for them.

Probably the biggest resistance to self-care is being told—and believing—that a condition can't be improved. Negative words about our health are powerful and become a medical hex when they get stuck in our minds. "You have very bad spinal degenerative disease and there's nothing you can do about it. You're never going to get any better." "You have neck pain? That's just old age. Get used to it!" The medical hex is stuck in our minds, and we feel stuck with the pain—often leading us to continue our search for a magical fix.

Chronic pain can lead to compulsive relief seeking. Everywhere we look, we are inundated and targeted by retail marketers for miraculous pain relievers and medical devices. Just the other day I had a robo-call for an "amazing pain relieving back brace" available to me now at a very low cost! Pain makes us anxious and susceptible to being taken advantage of. People are willing to try anything for their chronic pain—except for self-care, that is often ignored and easily discounted.

Inertia can stop us from taking care of ourselves. We make our New Year's resolutions with the best intention, thinking that willpower alone can make changes. But research has shown that willpower only works for a short time. Like getting up to the top of a steep hill or going to the gym until mid January—but it can't help with long-term behavioral change. We often look for short cuts—the easiest way to get results. If things don't change quickly, we can become discouraged and just want to give up.

This is why taking a pill for pain relief is so appealing. We want to believe that they work. But for long-term relief of orthopedic pains, they really don't work. Worse than just not working, they're very harmful. And even worse than being told you need to take them, is then having them taken away from you. After so many tragic stories of addiction and overdose, opiates aren't given out so freely anymore. This is a good thing. But what will take their place? The American Physical Therapy Association (APTA) is raising awareness about the risks of opioids and the safe alternative of physical therapy.

We can let pain define us and we carry these identities with us— cultural histories, family histories, and personal histories of physical and emotional suffering. These memories can shape our beliefs in how we care for ourselves. Beliefs that we need to have stronger drugs. Beliefs that we need to have just one more surgery. Beliefs that we just haven't found the right someone to fix us.

What if we could step away from these identities? Step away from thoughts that hold us back and move beyond seeking a source of relief outside ourselves. Take a small step towards psychological and behavioral change, by understanding pain and becoming responsible for our own care where we can. Once we've had a successful direct experience with self-care, we can begin to have a new identity. Preventative care and education is key to improving health care outcomes. Emotions run high when we don't know what to do for our painful conditions.

It's Never Too Late

An elderly friend of mine had been diagnosed with lumbar degenerative joint and disc disease, and spinal stenosis 15 years ago. He would occasionally have flare-ups and would get an epidural injection to relieve his symptoms, and had a prescription for Vicodin. At first he needed an injection once a year, then twice a year. He was getting them about every 3 months, when a few years ago he weed whacked for three days in a row, severely straining his back. He had horrible back and sciatic pain and he needed to begin walking with a walker instead of using a cane. The doctor told him that he couldn't keep giving him injections—they weren't helping anymore—and that the only thing he could do was to take more Vicodin.

He began taking Vicodin every 4 hours—even waking up in the wee hours of the morning to take a pill. Getting his prescription had become more difficult with new medical guidelines for opiates. He said he felt like a criminal just getting his medication. He became less and less active. He wasn't able to take walks like he used to. He wasn't comfortable driving anymore.

This went on for two years. Then he had a medical emergency that landed him in the hospital. While in the hospital, he would be asked if he had any pain. The first night he said he did, and was given Norco. After that, he said he didn't need anything for pain. He was lying in bed and not getting up at all at the time. After a week in the hospital, he went into a nursing care center for a couple of weeks, and never asked for pain pills.

He got home, in a weakened state, and asked me "So, when do I start taking Vicodin again?" I told him that he didn't need to start taking it again. What he needed was to get stronger. "But my doctor prescribed it for me!" I explained that it was only for pain his doctor couldn't help him with otherwise. It wasn't for any medical condition and had serious side effects. He hadn't taken it for over a month and was doing well without it. Why would he want to start taking it again? He consulted his doctor and started taking over-the-counter acetaminophen instead, as needed.

I encouraged him to gradually do more to improve his strength. He took this to heart. I showed him PIL in sitting and standing. He started walking to his mailbox, at first having to sit and rest on his walker half way there and back. He had firewood delivered to his house. He started to stack it himself. It took him two weeks to stack the first load. A second load was delivered that he stacked in one week. After a while, he thought he'd try to drive his car a short distance. He felt so good that he decided to go all the way into the nearby town.

Now, it's a year later. He drives himself into town an hour away and is getting ready to have his driver's license renewed at age 88. He walks mostly without a cane, but carries it and uses it occasionally. He walks slightly bent forward, and still has occasional pain. But his quality of life is vastly improved since he got his strength back, started sleeping better, doing more—and stopped taking Vicodin!

We can start with timely self-care by being present—observing thoughts and emotional reactions to pain—or any other annoyance! Notice what thoughts pop up the next time we experience an acute pain, or when someone's bugging us. Awareness begins by observing thoughts and taking slow, deep breaths. Feel the calming effects as we focus on breathing. Then do PIL and continue to breathe slowly. That's all it takes to begin. Small steps.

Do PIL during the day—instead of taking a pill—and do Slump/ PIL at night and in the morning. Let any ache, pain, or stiffness be a reminder to do it. Practice mindful body awareness so it becomes second nature. Have an elastic exercise band around the house for when it's needed. If nothing else, don't forget where this book is!

Healthy aging means staying strong and active. The real magic we have is the body's innate ability to heal and regain strength throughout our lives.

"Be fully aware of what you're doing and work becomes the yoga of work, play becomes the yoga of play, everyday living becomes the yoga of everyday living."

—Aldous Huxley, *The Island*, 1962

Acknowledgements

Writing this book occurred in fits and starts. If I hadn't had the encouragement, urging, and help of many people along the way it would never have been completed. I thank you all.

I'll start by thanking the hundreds of people I've seen over the years who have entrusted me with their stories along with their bodies. What I have taught you, you have taught me more.

Gratitude goes out to Mary Radu, a writer and client whom I first shared my idea for this book. Her enthusiasm for the concept and her enjoyment of my way of explaining PT principles in an easy to understand manner, gave me the first inkling that I could actually write a book. Little did I know what I was in for—the time and work it would take! How hard could it be? Ignorance was definitely blissful.

In the early stage of this process, thanks to Mary DeDanan for her editing, and kind and gentle prodding to finish the first draft. Cheers to Stephanie Endsley for our fun with artistic collaboration. Thanks again to Mary Radu and my PT buddies Dave Sereni and Camilla Cinquini for reading through my first stream of consciousness draft and for letting me know I was on the right track. Special thanks to Jody Trock for honestly letting me know it needed a lot of work, starting me on the journey of several rewrites.

Appreciation goes out to Caroline Paul and Canyon Sam, published authors and friends, to hear my pitch and give me advice and recommendations. I was referred to Joan Gelfund, a writing coach, who pushed me to pitch it to publishers and connected me to Daniella Granados for her web page and marketing skills. Thanks to you both.

PT buddy Bernie Guth has been an inspiration and mystical guide throughout my career, exploring the deeper side of physical therapy by being skeptical while keeping a sense of humor. Your help with Part One of the book was invaluable.

My crew of final proofreaders/editors is especially near and dear to my heart. All contributed a different angle on the finishing touches of the final rewrite. Sylvia Murphy, really got the spirit of the book and helped so much with the introduction; Marion Schoenfeld—thanks for the Em dashes and all the other punctuation help I needed and correcting my many boo boos; and Gretchen Butler, who went above and beyond anything I could have expected with editing.

Thanks to Joop Delahaye (also a PT buddy) and his wife Nancy Schwartz for dropping by on the day I needed to find someone to help me with illustrations. They just happened to have a very good friend who fit the bill. Gary Newman has been the best Photoshop manipulator and illustrator I could have hoped for, who then stepped up to do the layout and final proof reading. It's been a joy to work with you, Gary.

Most of all, I thank my wife Gayle. Not just for pointing out how much I used "a bit" in my original draft and helping with the epilogue, but for being solid when I faltered on my resolve and who keeps me directed toward joyfulness in our pursuit of awareness. There is no opposite of love.

References

Begley, Sharon. *Train Your Mind, Change Your Brain.* New York: Ballantine Books, 2007.

Butler, David, and Moseley, G. Lorimer. *Explain Pain.* Australia, NOI Group Publication, 2003.

Chopra, Deepak, MD. *Ageless Body, Timeless Mind.* New York: Harmony Books, 1993.

Darnall, Beth, PhD. *Less Pain, Fewer Pills: Avoid the Dangers of Prescription Opioids and Gain Control Over Chronic Pain.* Boulder, CO: Bull Publishing Company, 2014.

Gifford, Louis. *Aches and Pains.* Kestrel, Swanpool, Falmouth, Cornwall, UK: CNS Press, 2014.

Jakobson Ramin, Cathryn. *Crooked: Outwitting The Back Pain Industry and Getting On The Road To Recovery.* New York: Harper Collins, 2017.

Kabat-Zinn, Jon. *Full Catastrophe Living.* New York: Bantan Books, 1990.

Kabat-Zinn, Jon. *The Healing Power of Mindfulness: A New Way of Being.* Hachette Books, 2018.

King, Brian, PhD. *How The Brain Forms New Habits: Why Willpower is Not Enough.* Lecture through the Institute for Brain Potential, 2012.

Louw Adriaan, PT, PhD, CSMT. *Why Do I Hurt? A Patient Book About the Neuroscience of Pain.* USA: International Spine and Pain Institute, 2013.

Melzack, Ronald and Wall, Patrick. *The Challenge of Pain.* Middlesex, England: Penguin Books, 1982.

Sieber, Bill, PhD. *Listening to the Body: Understanding The Language of Stress Related Symptoms.* Lecture/DVD through the Institute for Brain Potential, 2014.

William and Warwick. *Gray's Anatomy.* 36th British Edition, Philadelphia: WB Saunders Company, 1980.

About the Author

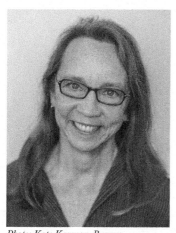

Photo: Kate Karwan-Burgess

Wanda Swenson has been a physical therapist for over 30 years. She received her education at San Francisco State University and received her Physical Therapy degree from the University of California at San Francisco in 1986.

She began working at Kaiser Permanente Oakland, CA outpatient department in 1988. After moving to Sonoma County in 1993, she worked at Kaiser Permanente Santa Rosa, CA, becoming a clinical instructor in addition to treating patients individually and teaching classes. She is a member of the APTA.

Retiring from Kaiser Permanente in 2013, she continues to practice physical therapy in her rural community in the coastal hills of Sonoma County, where she and her wife Gayle live and tend an olive grove to produce olive oil. Writing her first book, she brings together her life long interest in eastern philosophies and mind body awareness, with her dedication to physical therapy in her *"How Of Ow"* approach to self-care.